The MRI Practitioner's Handbook
Essential Safety and Scanning Information

Barbara Nugent

Class Professional Publishing have made every effort to ensure that the information, tables, drawings and diagrams contained in this book are accurate at the time of publication. The book cannot always contain all the information necessary for determining appropriate care and cannot address all individual situations; therefore, individuals using the book must ensure they have the appropriate knowledge and skills to enable suitable interpretation. Class Professional Publishing does not guarantee, and accepts no legal liability of whatever nature arising from or connected to, the accuracy, reliability, currency or completeness of the content of *The MRI Practitioner's Handbook: Essential Safety and Scanning Information*. Users must always be aware that such innovations or alterations after the date of publication may not be incorporated in the content. Please note, however, that Class Professional Publishing assumes no responsibility whatsoever for the content of external resources in the text or accompanying online materials.

Text © Barbara Nugent

All rights reserved. Without limiting the rights under copyright reserved above, no part of this publication may be reproduced, stored in or introduced into a retrieval system, or transmitted, in any form or by any means (electronic, mechanical, photocopying, recording or otherwise) without the prior written permission of the publisher of this book.

The information presented in this book is accurate and current to the best of the authors' knowledge. The authors and publisher, however, make no guarantee as to, and assume no responsibility for, the correctness, sufficiency or completeness of such information or any recommendations. Any recommendations or views expressed in this handbook represent the opinion of the author.

Printing history

This edition first printed in 2024; updated and reprinted in 2024
The authors and publisher welcome feedback from the users of this book.

Please contact the publisher:

Class Professional Publishing,
The Exchange, Express Park, Bristol Road, Bridgwater TA6 4RR

Telephone: 01278 472 800
Email: info@class.co.uk
Website: www.classprofessional.co.uk

Class Professional Publishing is an imprint of Class Publishing Ltd
A CIP catalogue record for this book is available from the British Library

Paperback ISBN: 9781801611190
Cover design by Nicky Borowiec

Designed and typeset by PHi Business Solutions
Printed in the UK by Hobbs

This book is printed on paper from responsible sources. Refer to local recycling guidance on disposal of this book.

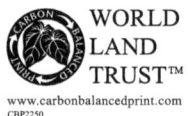

If found, please return this handbook to:
Name:
Location:
Contact Details:

Table of Contents

Acknowledgements ... ix
About MRI Safety Matters ... xi
About the Author ... xi
How to Use This Handbook ... xiii
Seeking Safety Guidance in Your Organisation ... xv
List of Acronyms and Abbreviations ... xvii

1 Contact Information ... 1
Table 1.1   MRI Safety Leads, Service or Department Contact Information ... 1
Table 1.2   Equipment, Device, Manufacturer or Vendor Contact Information ... 2

2 MRI Safety Information ... 3
MR Controlled Access Areas and Safety Zones ... 3
Table 2.1   Typical Department Restricted Areas/Zoning System ... 3
Figure 2.1 Depiction of a Typical MR Controlled Access Area (CAA) Showing the MHRA and the ACR Area Descriptions ... 4
Table 2.2   Patient Screening Factors to Consider ... 4
Table 2.3   Safety Processes to Consider, Post-Screening ... 9

Labelling Items for MR Safety Conditions of Use ... 12
The Definitions and Labelling used for Marking Equipment Taken Into the MR Environment ... 12
Figure 2.2 Definitions from ASTM International Standard F2503-13 ... 12

MR Conditions of Use ... 12
MR Conditional Labelling to Indicate the Conditions of Use in the MR Environment ... 13
Figure 2.3 Examples of MR Conditional Labelling and an MR Unsafe Label ... 13

MRI Department Safety Signage ... 13
Figure 2.4 Examples of Safety Signage from IPEM ... 13

Considerations to Prevent Patient Burns and Overheating ... 14
Table 2.4   Considerations to Prevent Patient Burns and Overheating ... 14

Understanding SAR and B1+rms ... 20
Table 2.5   Typical High and Low SAR Pulse Sequences ... 21
Table 2.6   Considerations to Reduce SAR ... 22

Mode of Operation Considerations ... 23
Table 2.7   Standards for Modes of Operation ... 23

Static Magnetic Fields ... 24
Table 2.8   Mode of Operation Considerations: Static Magnetic Fields (B_0) ... 25

Time-varying Magnetic Field Gradients ... 25
Table 2.9   Mode of Operation Considerations: Time-varying Magnetic Field Gradients (dB/dt) ... 25

RF Magnetic Fields (B_1) ... 25
Table 2.10 RF Magnetic Fields (B_1) ... 25

Weight and Height Measurement Conversion Charts		26
Weight Measurement Conversion Chart		26
Height Measurement Conversion Chart		27
Considerations for Managing Implants		28
Table 2.11	Passive and Active Implant Descriptions	28
Infographic 2.1	Stages of a Typical MRI Appointment	29
Infographic 2.2	Stages of a Typical Implant or FB Investigation	30
Table 2.12	Template for Logging the Procedures for Dealing with Passive Implants	31
Table 2.13	Template for Logging the Procedures for Dealing with Active Implants	32
Unlabelled Devices/Implants		33
Table 2.14	Template for Logging the Procedures for Dealing with Unlabelled Devices/Implants	33
Procedure for Dealing with Unlabelled Devices/Implants		35
Table 2.15	Template to Record Implant/Device Information (× 6)	36

3 Equipment Information — 43

Table 3.1	Some Suggested Regular and Planned Checks to Consider	43
Table 3.2	Considerations When Scanning QA/QC Phantom(s)	47
Table 3.3	Post-Scanning Considerations: QA/QC Phantom(s)	47
Table 3.4	Template for Recording Specific Scanner Information (× 6)	48
Table 3.5	A Typical Equipment Repair and Maintenance Records Template	54
Table 3.6	Names and Types of Coils	55
Infographic 3.1	Compliant Coil Labelling	56

4 Pulse Sequence Information and Considerations — 59

Table 4.1	Template for Recording Pulse Sequence Parameters and Information	59
Table 4.1a	Template for Recording Protocol Information	60
Table 4.2	Template for Noting Scanner Manufacturers' Pulse Sequence Terminology	61
Table 4.3	Pulse Sequence Parameter Trade-Offs	62
Table 4.4	General Considerations When Planning Slices and Sequences	63

5 Preparing for Emergency Situations — 67

Standard Operating Procedures for Dealing with Emergencies		67
Table 5.1	Examples of Scenarios	67
Some General Considerations When Dealing with Emergencies and Urgent Situations in an MRI Department		70

6 Developing a Protocol for MRI Safety Checks During General Anaesthetic (GA) MRI Sessions — 73

Figure 6.1	Some Checks to Consider Before the Patient is Called to the Department	74
Figure 6.2	Some Checks and Pauses to Consider When the Patient Arrives at the MRI Department	75
Table 6.1	Further Considerations for MRI GA Sessions – Notes	76

7 Infection Control Processes — 79

Table 7.1	Infection Prevention and Control Considerations/Notes	79

8 Templates for Recording Protocol Information — 83

Table 8.1	Protocol Table Template (× 3)	83
Table 8.1a	Preparations (× 3)	84
Table 8.2	Emergency Spine Protocol	89
Table 8.2a	Emergency Spine Imaging Preparations	90
Table 8.3	Neuro/Brain Protocol	91
Table 8.3a	Neuro/Brain Imaging Preparations	92
Table 8.4	Musculoskeletal Protocol Table	93
Table 8.4a	Musculoskeletal Imaging Preparations	94
Table 8.5	Angiography Protocol	95
Table 8.5a	Angiography Imaging Preparations	96
Table 8.6	Liver Protocol	97
Table 8.6a	Liver Imaging Preparations	98
Table 8.7	Small Bowel Imaging/Enterography Protocol	99
Table 8.7a	Small Bowel/Enterography Imaging Preparations	100
Table 8.8	Breast Imaging Protocol	101
Table 8.8a	Breast Imaging Preparations	102
Table 8.9	Prostate Imaging Protocol	103
Table 8.9a	Prostate Imaging Preparations	104
Table 8.10	Cardiac Imaging Protocol	105
Table 8.10a	Cardiac Imaging Preparations	106
Table 8.11	Whole Body Imaging Protocol	107
Table 8.11a	Whole Body Imaging Preparations	108
Table 8.12	Paediatric Imaging Protocol (× 4)	109
Table 8.12a	Paediatric Imaging Preparations (× 4)	110
Table 8.13	Active Research Projects Protocols	117
Table 8.13a	Active Research Projects Preparations	118
Table 8.14	Escalation Process If Pathology Seen	119

9 Contrast Considerations — 121

Table 9.1	Adverse Contrast/Drug Reaction Considerations	121
Table 9.2	eGFR and Creatinine Notes	122
Table 9.3	Contrast Injection Considerations for Patients with Additional Needs	122
Table 9.4	Other Processes to Consider	123
Table 9.5	Template of Contrast or Other Drug Administration Notes (× 6)	124

10 Image Artefact Considerations — 131

Figure 10.1	Depiction of Typical MRI Image Artefacts	131

11 Miscellaneous Topics and Concerns — 133

Figure 11.1	Managing a Stressful List	133
Table 11.1	Additional Topics to Consider	134

12 Recording Continuing Professional Development (CPD) — 139

Table 12.1	A Template to Note CPD Activities	140

13 Resources — 143

Acknowledgements

The author is indebted to the following individuals for either contributing to or reviewing parts of this handbook, or reviewing and/or contributing to its forerunner, which was called the 'MRI Operator Notebook' (designed for UK/European MRI Operators). The author sincerely thanks every one of these MRI professionals for supporting the need for this project and for providing their considered opinion and suggestions for the type of content to include.

Listed in Alphabetical Order by First Name

Alex Shcherbakov (ARRT) (R) (MR) CRT SCRQSA
Alison Gwynne Davies DCR (R) PG DMS
Avinash Kanodia MBBS MD DM FRCR MRMD (MRSC™)
Catherine Westbrook EdD MSc DCR(R) CTC
Darren Hudson BSc (Hons) MHSc PgCert MRSO (MRSC™)
David Grainger MSc MIPEM
David Hewson BSc (Hons) MSc MRSO (MRSC™)
Elisabeth Ioele Bsc (Hons) PgC (MRI) MRSO (MRSC™)
Elizabeth Ashburner BSc (Hons)
Elizabeth Squire HDCR MRSO (MRSC™)
Helen Estall MSc AFHEA BSc (Hons) DCR(R)
Ian Cavin BSc (Hons) MSc PhD SRCS MRSE (MRSC™)
Ivor Lobel DCR(R) PgC (MRI)
James Berry BSc (Hons)
Johnathan Hewis MSc Med Imag PgCert LTHE PgCert BE BSc Hons DiRad FHEA
Jonathan Ashmore BSc (Hons) MSc PhD CSci
Karen Smith DCR(R) PgC MRSO (MRSC™)
Lisa Serevena Bsc (Hons) BA (Hons) CMgr MCMI
Mark Johnson BSc MSc PgD (MRI Reporting)
Martin J. Graves PhD CSci MIET MRCR(Hon) FHEA FIPEM FISMRM FBIR MRSE (MRSC™)
Pam Mitchell DCR(R) MRSO (MRSC™)
Rachel Watt MSc BSc
Rebecca Magrath BSc (Hons) MRSO (MRSC™)
Rhys Slough MSc BSc (Hons)
Samuel Oliveira Bsc (Hons) PgD MRSO (MRSC™)
Sohail Bhana MSc MRSO (MRSC™)
Sonya Castle BSc (Hons)
Susan Murch DCR(R) MRSO (MRSC™)
Tobias Gilk MArch, MRSO (MRSC™), MRSE (MRSC™)
Wendy Milne DCR(R)

Special thanks to Elizabeth Ashburner for allowing the author to modify two infographics. The author is also especially grateful to Professor Martin J. Graves, Helen Estall and Rachel Watt for their assistance and for providing their time and expertise to review some of the material.

I would also like to thank my husband, Keith Nugent, for all his support.

This handbook evolved from many contributions and suggestions from highly experienced and qualified MRI professionals. Their unwavering commitment to advancing MRI education, dedication to their profession and to learning are inspirational and without their generosity of spirit and support, this resource would not have been possible.

The author would also like to sincerely thank Alex Shcherbakov (ARRT) (R) (MR) CRT SCRQSA of Scanmate.co for his support and encouragement, and for collaborating on an earlier resource which provided the inspiration for development of this handbook. Alex created a customised notebook containing templates designed to record relevant MRI information with ease. Some of the templates contained within this resource are modified from that earlier collaborative project. Alex's 'MRI Operator Notebook' can be found at Scanmate.co.

About MRI Safety Matters®

The aims of MRI Safety Matters® are to develop, expand and share MRI safety knowledge with the MRI community and to foster national and global collaborations to progress MRI safety initiatives.Through training events, we provide opportunities to learn from experts and peers and to network with industry partners.

MRI Safety Matters® runs Kanal's European MRMD/MRSO course and an annual hybrid MRI Safety Update and Innovation conference. We have twice hosted the ABMRS to administer UK-modified MRI safety exams (MRSO, MRMD and MRSE), leading to the first two cohorts of ABMRS MR safety credentialled Radiographers, Radiologists, Physicists and Clinical Scientists in Europe. For more information, please visit mrisafetymatters.com

https://www.mrisafetymatters.co.uk/

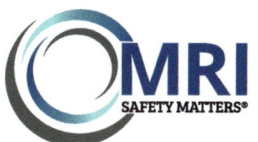

About the Author

Barbara Nugent
BSC(Hons) DCR(R) PGC(MRI) MRSO(MRSC™) MIPEM

Barbara is a former MRI and CT Superintendent Radiographer, and was an MRI safety project lead for NHS National Education for Scotland. She is a visiting lecturer at City, University of London, and has been a subject matter specialist for several companies. As the founder of MRI Safety Matters®, Barbara's main aims are to promote MRI safety initiatives and education, and to advocate for MRI staff to be provided with a recognised standard of MRI safety knowledge.

As part of a UK multi-professional working group, Barbara has been involved in developing a programme of national e-learning modules for those that work in MRI and those whose role is associated with MRI.

How to Use This Handbook

The specific templates and colour-coded sections have been carefully designed to provide a simple way for you to store and find MRI scanning and safety information and to organise appropriate work-related notes. Some topics and processes to consider when developing local guidance and SOPs are suggested but your department's agreed local guidance and processes are to be followed. SOPs should detail local procedures, adhering to relevant national and professional bodies' regulations and advice.

Please do not use this resource to store any confidential, personal or patient-related information and always keep your information current.

This handbook is designed for personal use but it is envisaged that the content may serve to assist departments to consider what content they might require when developing their local policies and procedures.

Seeking Safety Guidance in Your Organisation

Please note that for information on MRI safety practices, always follow your department local rules, guidance and SOPs. MRI safety guidance is available from your organisation as well as from professional and regulatory bodies.

This handbook is aimed at MRI Practitioners who follow MHRA guidance (Magnetic Resonance Imaging Equipment in Clinical Use: Safety Guidelines). It is recommended to always follow guidance from the latest version of your regulator's safety guidance as well as from your professional body.

For information to guide the decision to scan medically implanted devices, follow your local guidance or SOPs. You can access the latest safety information about implants/devices through the relevant manufacturer's website or by contacting the manufacturer directly.

Know who to contact locally within your organisation for guidance regarding safety issues. If you are not involved with the local MR Safety Committee, you could find out who is and how to contact those who can assist with any MR safety-related concerns. It may prove useful to know, for example, who the managers for MRI safety are in your organisation, including the MR Responsible Person (normally the Lead Radiographer), the Lead Radiologist, the MRSO (if one is assigned), and the MRSE. An MRSE has an advanced knowledge of MRI techniques and an appropriate understanding of the clinical applications of MRI to provide scientific advice for assessing MR conditions of use for certain implants and devices and may provide advice when developing MRI safety protocols and SOPs.

One of the roles of a departmental or regional MRSO, who is usually a highly experienced and knowledgeable MR Radiographer, is to assist with MRI safety-related activities and processes. For more information about an MRSO role, please see the Resources section.

Feedback

We would appreciate any feedback on this handbook to identify any content you would like to see in future editions. Please contact us at hello@mrisafetymatters.co.uk

Disclaimer

No warranties of any kind are declared or implied in the contents. Readers acknowledge that the author is not engaging in the rendering of technical, medical or professional advice. Under no circumstances is the author responsible for any losses, direct or indirect, which are incurred because of the use of the information contained within this handbook, including but not limited to errors, omissions, or inaccuracies.

List of Acronyms and Abbreviations

ABMRS	American Board of Magnetic Resonance Safety | https://abmrs.org
ACR	American College of Radiology | https://www.acr.org/Clinical-Resources/Radiology-Safety/MR-Safety
ASTM	American Society for Testing and Materials. [International standards organisation that develops and publishes voluntary consensus technical standards for a wide range of materials, products, systems, and services] | https://www.astm.org/f2503-20.html
AXREM	Trade association representing suppliers of diagnostic medical imaging, radiotherapy, healthcare IT and care equipment in the UK | https://www.axrem.org.uk/
B_0	Static magnetic field
B1+rms	Root mean square of the RF magnetic field (B1) used for excitation which is averaged over a 10-second period
CAA	Controlled Access Area
CCTV	Closed-Circuit Television
CIED	Cardiac Implantable Electronic Device
CGM	Continuous Glucose Monitoring
CPD	Continuing Professional Development
CT	Computed Tomography
DoLS	Deprivation of Liberty Safeguards
ECG	Electrocardiogram
eGFR	estimated Glomerular Filtration Rate
EMF	Electromagnetic Field
ETL	Echo Train Length
FASE	Fast Advanced Spin Echo
FB	Foreign Body
FOV	Field of View
FMD	Ferromagnetic Detector
FSE	Fast Spin Echo
GA	General Anaesthetic
GISP	Generic Implant Safety Procedures (or Policies)
GRE	Gradient Echo
HASTE	Half-Fourier Acquisition Single-shot Turbo Spin Echo
HPA	Health Protection Agency
HOD	Head of Department
ICNRP	International Commission on Non-ionizing Radiation Protection | https://www.icnirp.org/en/publications/article/rf-guidelines-2020.html
IEC	International Electrotechnical Commission | https://www.iec.ch/government-regulators/medical-devices
IOFB	Intraorbital Foreign Body
IVC Filter	Inferior Vena Cava filter
IUD	Intrauterine Device
MHRA	Medicines and Healthcare products Regulatory Agency | https://www.gov.uk/government/publications/safety-guidelines-for-magnetic-resonance-imaging-equipment-in-clinical-use

MR ENVIRONMENT		'The three-dimensional volume of space surrounding the MR magnet that contains both the Faraday shielded volume and the 0.50 mT field contour gauss (G) line). This volume is the region in which an item might pose a hazard from exposure to the electromagnetic fields produced by the MR equipment and accessories.' (From MHRA MRI guidelines sec. 4.5.1 Definition of MR ENVIRONMENT as defined by the ASTM.)
MRI		Magnetic Resonance Imaging
MRMD		Magnetic Resonance Medical Director: Person who is operationally responsible for the MR facility, usually a medical doctor.
MR Operator		An MR Authorised Person who is a suitably trained member of staff authorised to have access to the MR CAA, one who is also entitled to operate the MRI equipment, normally radiographers or radiologists but may include assistant practitioners, physicists, maintenance and research staff). https://www.gov.uk/government/publications/safety-guidelines-for-magnetic-resonance-imaging-equipment-in-clinical-use
MR Projectile Zone		A locally defined volume which contains the full extent of the 3 mT magnetic field contour, or other appropriate measure, around the MRI scanner
MR Responsible Person		Person responsible for ensuring adequate written safety and emergency procedures and work and operating instructions are issued to appropriate staff, after full consultation with the MRSE and representatives of all MR Authorised Personnel. Delegated with the day-to-day responsibility for MR safety. https://www.gov.uk/government/publications/safety-guidelines-for-magnetic-resonance-imaging-equipment-in-clinical-use
MRSE		Magnetic Resonance Safety Expert: Designated professional who has an advanced knowledge of MRI techniques and an appropriate understanding of the clinical applications of MRI. Provides scientific advice to the MR Responsible Person. Role often undertaken by a Medical Physicist with expertise in MRI. https://www.gov.uk/government/publications/safety-guidelines-for-magnetic-resonance-imaging-equipment-in-clinical-use
MRSO		Magnetic Resonance Safety Officer: Responsible for executing the MR safety practices as defined/ordered for the site. Learn more about MRSO, MRSE and MRMD roles and exams at: https://www.acr.org/Clinical-Resources/Radiology-Safety/MR-Safety, https://abmrs.org/choosing-the-right-certification-type-for-you/, https://www.ipem.ac.uk/learn/cpd-and-post-registration-learning/mrse-certificate-of-competence/, and https://api.efrs.eu/api/assets/posts/256
NEX		Number of Excitations
NSA		Number of Signal Averages
PNS		Peripheral Nerve Stimulation
QA		Quality Assurance
QC		Quality Control
RF		Radio Frequency
RFID		Radio Frequency Identification
SAR		Specific Absorption Rate
SE		Spin Echo
SNR		Signal to Noise Ratio
SOP		Standard Operating Procedure	https://learn.nes.nhs.scot/30397
SS-FSE		Single Shot Fast Spin-Echo
SSH-TSE		Single-Shot Turbo Spin-Echo
TE		Time to Echo
TR		Repetition Time
TSE		Turbo Spin Echo

1 Contact Information

Table 1.1 MRI Safety Leads, Service or Department Contact Information

MRI Safety Leads	Contact Information (For confidentiality purposes, be discreet, e.g. use only initials or a first name, where appropriate)	Notes
MR Responsible Person		
MRSO		
MRSE		
HOD		
Lead Radiologist		
Service or Department		

Table 1.2 Equipment, Device, Manufacturer or Vendor Contact Information

Equipment or Device	Contact Information	Notes
Manufacturer or Vendor		

2 MRI Safety Information

MR Controlled Access Areas and Safety Zones

Table 2.1 Typical Department Restricted Areas/Zoning System

Depiction of a typical MR CAA showing examples of the types of set up that might exist for each area with corresponding MHRA Controlled Access Areas and suggested ACR Zones. Please note that ACR zones are not specifically tied to all the MRI suite rooms or functions. They are, instead, designed to map the areas of MR risk and function. It is only Zone 4 that the ACR specifically associates with a room, the MRI Scanner/Magnet Room. All other ACR Zones are indications of risks, regardless of which rooms / functions they include.

MRI Areas	Zone 1 (ACR)	Zone 2 (ACR)	MR CAA (MHRA) Zone 3 (ACR)	MR Environment (MHRA) Zone 4 (ACR)
Typical CAAs and MRI Safety Zone layouts	Zone 1	Zone 2	CAA/Zone 3	MR Environment/ Zone 4
Examples of the types of layout of each area. Please note that variations exist.	Zone 1 space has neither MRI risk nor MRI function. These are areas that are unrestricted and freely accessible to the public outside of the MRI department. This is not an area classified by the MHRA.	Interface between publicly accessible and unrestricted access areas (Zone 1) and CAAs. This is an area that has an MRI function (e.g., reception, waiting, changing rooms, interview areas, patient transfer areas etc.) but in which there is no persistent MRI-specific risk. This is not an area classified by the MHRA.	A locally defined area of such a size to contain the MR ENVIRONMENT. Access shall be restricted and suitable warning signs should be displayed at all entrances (MHRA). Zone 3 (ACR) is considered to be an area that has either or both a persistent MR risk (i.e., 0.5 mT /0.9 mT regions), and / or has direct physical access to Zone 4. As per local design, this area might contain rooms for various functions e.g. the control room and final checking area (with direct access to Zone 4) and the technical/ equipment room (which might, for example, be exposed to the 0.5 mT / 0.9 mT regions).	MR Environment – three-dimensional volume surrounding the magnet, contains the Faraday shielded volume and the 0.50 mT field contour, a region in which an item might pose a hazard from exposure to the EMFs produced by the magnet and accessories (ASTM). Contains the MR Projectile Zone – locally defined volume containing the full extent of the 3 mT magnetic field contour, or other appropriate measure, around the scanner (MHRA). Zone 4 – scanner/magnet room - contains the projectile risk and potential for exposure to time varying gradient and RF risks.

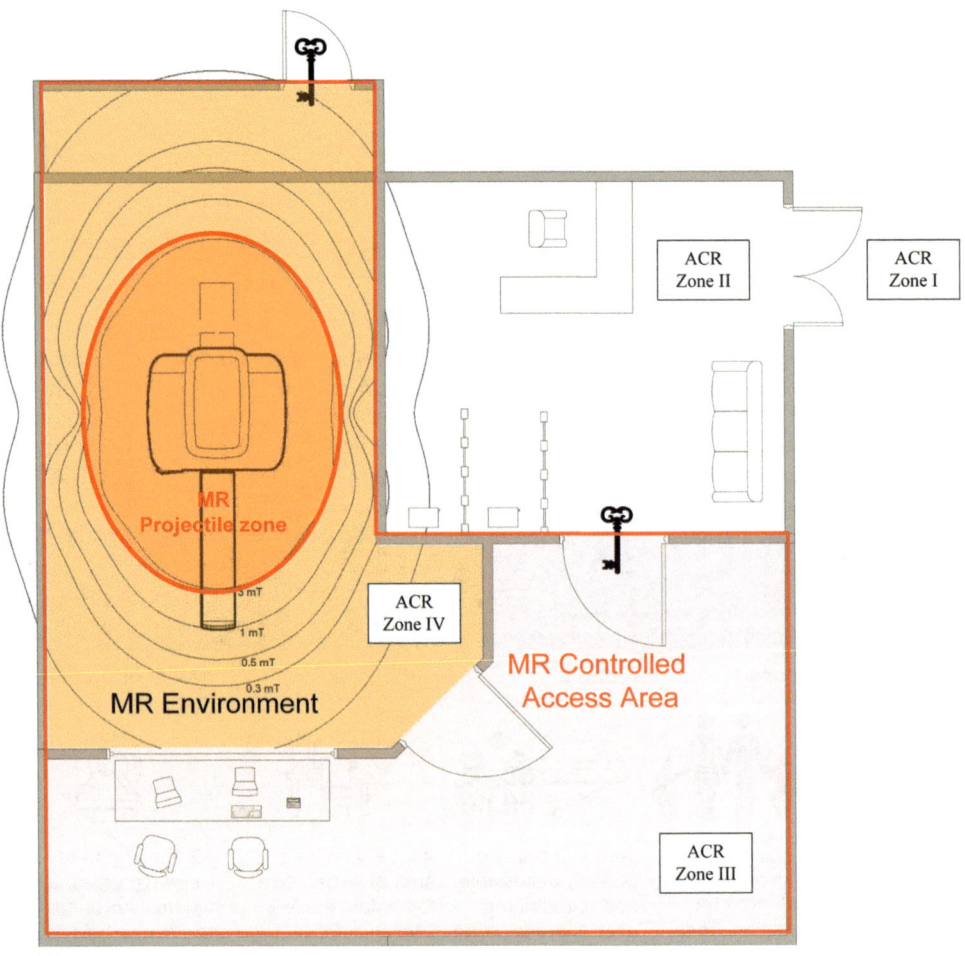

Figure 2.1 Depiction of a Typical MR CAA Showing the MHRA and ACR Area Descriptions.
Reproduced with permission of the MHRA under the terms of the Open Government Licence (OGL) v3.0

From MHRA 4.4.1 Definition of MR CONTROLLED ACCESS AREA

Table 2.2 Patient Screening Factors to Consider

Patient Screening Factors to Consider	Considerations	Notes
Screening form	Is it user friendly, i.e. written in plain language and a format that is easy to read?	
	What languages is it available in?	
	Has a lay person had input into the questions asked and format?	
	If it's an electronic form, is this a suitable format for all users, e.g. those with learning difficulties or those not familiar with filling in forms electronically?	

Patient Screening Factors to Consider	Considerations	Notes
	Are sufficient and appropriate questions being asked? Does it include, for example, asking if they have swallowed a pill camera (capsule endoscopy)?	
	Is there a standardised document that the questions are being sourced from?	
	Have you considered including the question: is there anything in, or on, your body that you were not born with?	
	Does it include alternating questions that require 'yes' or 'no' answers to try to ensure that each question is being carefully read and understood?	
	If the patient is sent the questionnaire, and they say 'yes' to key questions, indicating that they have possible MRI contraindications (a pacemaker, for example), does the form provide details of the appropriate department to contact to discuss further? This could clarify the situation to better manage the patient's booking.	
	Are there screening forms specifically designed for appropriate questioning of staff, visitors and volunteer patients?	
	Have readability/document design assessment tools been used to ensure the design and content of the questionnaire is appropriate?	
	Is there a translation service available, e.g. a language phoneline or local translator?	
	Other than written checks, what verbal and visual checks are performed before permitting anyone entry to the scan room?	
	Are there specific risk assessment forms for checking implants, devices, or foreign bodies? If so, who undertakes the assessment and signs off this form?	
	Who is permitted to countersign the screening form to state that the patient is safe to scan, bearing in mind that the screening form is a medico-legal document?	
	The signed screening form becomes part of the patient's medical record. How long is the screening form held for in your organisation and where are the completed screening forms securely stored?	

(Continued)

MRI Safety Information

Patient Screening Factors to Consider	Considerations	Notes
Consent	What are the types of patient consent that exist and when can they be used?	
	How do you know if you are receiving true consent from cognitive patients?	
	How do you ensure your patients understand the questions you are asking them?	
	If a referring clinician is urging that an MRI scan on their patient should be done but the patient is unable to consent for their scan, what safeguards are in place for those deemed not to have capacity to consent? (See Resources section for information on DoLS.)	
	Regulations play a crucial role in safeguarding vulnerable individuals who cannot consent to their care and treatment. How are you made familiar with safeguarding regulations? Is it part of mandatory training?	
	Is there a written policy to follow if a translation service is used to gain consent from a patient? Does local guidance or a SOP detail how consent is achieved using a translation service and who is allowed to translate?	
Patient clothing	Is your local policy to change patients into a hospital gown or scrubs? Has your dept. considered using pocketless patient clothing with long sleeves and trousers to try to prevent limbs from touching bare skin? Having no pockets could prevent hidden items from inadvertently entering the scan room. For the purposes of dignity, some patients might prefer to wear scrub trousers.	
	Clothing labelling does not always mention the presence of metal fibres or metal treatments (e.g. technology in some sports clothing and underwear).	
	Has your dept. considered asking patients to remove certain clothing to prevent this and are they provided with appropriate MR safe alternatives if that part of their anatomy will be exposed to the RF?	
Methods to identify ferromagnetic and non-ferromagnetic items on a patient	How can you identify metallic items on, or in, a patient?	
	What processes are in place to detect ferromagnetic and non-ferromagnetic metallic items?	
	Is there a process to follow to check if any metallic items that cannot be removed from the patient are magnetic i.e. ferrous? If a ferromagnetic detector or an appropriate hand held detector, for example, is used, is there local guidance on their use and function?	

Patient Screening Factors to Consider	Considerations	Notes
	FMDs are intended as an additional screening tool to identify ferrous items. They do not detect all metallic objects. Consider where and how any tool used for detecting metallic items are to be used to ensure the process is performed in a safe place, in a safe way and the process is understood..	
	If you see susceptibility artefact (signal void) on an image, this could be caused by metal. Pause or stop the sequence to investigate and remove the cause.	
Jewellery and wearable technology policy	What is the local policy when a patient's jewellery or dermal piercing cannot easily be removed?	
	If manufacturer guidelines cannot be followed for safe scanning of patients with wearable technologies such as health and fitness trackers and CGMs, is there a policy to follow for such devices? For patients who wear CGMs, consider booking their appointment when their device is due to be replaced and providing information to this effect in pre-appointment information.	
	Information regarding any drug/dermal patches could be mentioned in the patient pr-appointment information too so that patients are aware of the department's removal policy and come prepared by bringing a replacement patch, if required.	
Screening non-cognitive patients	Is there an SOP to follow when a patient is unable to complete their safety questionnaire?	
	What methods are used to ensure the patient has no contraindicated implants? What constitutes appropriate/reliable evidence for screening purposes, e.g. clinician's advice, medical records, visual inspection, use of FMD/handheld detectors, recent imaging, etc.? What is the sign-off process and who is considered the appropriate person to investigate and state that the patient is safe to scan or not?	
	Where necessary, what diagnostic imaging is undertaken to try to identify if the patient has contraindicated implants or foreign bodies? (E.g. skull, chest and abdominal X-rays, or alternative imaging?)	
Performing implant/device/foreign body checks	Are there written procedures to follow that provide instructions on how to investigate implants, devices and foreign bodies?	
	What is the process for further investigation and who can be sought for further advice?	
	Is there a training and sign-off process for those that may assist with the process of checking implants and relevant scanning conditions e.g. the MR Responsible Person and/or MRSO?	

(Continued)

Patient Screening Factors to Consider	Considerations	Notes
Patient suitability	If the patient is very large, how is their girth checked to see if they will safely fit into the scanner, or their weight checked if they are too heavy for conventional scales? Is there a suitable measuring tape, and what is the width of the scanner? Is there an agreed policy of the words to use to ask the patient about their weight and girth to ensure sensitivity (so as not to inadvertently upset the patient)? Is there an agreed, easily remembered phrase to sensitively inform the patient that they are too large or heavy to be scanned? Who can you call on if the process of trying to explain the situation to the patient becomes too difficult? Would it be worth considering procuring a plastic hoop that could demonstrate to patients, where appropriate, the diameter/width of the bore? If so, and if necessary, could you develop a protocol that describes a sensitive way to ask the patient if they will allow you to see if they will first fit in such a hoop before putting them in the scanner bore? What is the maximum weight the scanner table and ancillary equipment, e.g. the patient retrieval MR Conditional trolley or MR Conditional wheelchair, can carry? Are there alternatives to suggest to the patient if the patient is not suitable to be scanned in that scanner? Can they be referred to a department which has a wider bore scanner or to an alternative imaging modality, for example? Is there a process to follow for informing the referrer if the patient is not suitable to be scanned?	
Accountability	Points to consider which may help to define responsibilities or accountability for safety: • Who is considered responsible for the patient's safety while the patient is in the scan room? • What responsibility does the person turning on the electromagnetic fields, performing the scan, starting the pump injector, etc. have? • What is the responsibility of the person who countersigned the screening form to say the patient was safe to scan? • What is the responsibility of the person taking the patient into the scan room? • What is the responsibility of the supervising radiologist or person supervising the scan?	

MRI Safety Information

Patient Screening Factors to Consider	Considerations	Notes
	• Several people may be involved in the many tasks associated with the patient's appointment, e.g. screening the patient, cannulating the patient, checking, and flushing the cannula, filling the pump, drawing up contrast or other relevant drugs, positioning the patient in the scanner and positioning patient padding, etc. How is appropriate communication between all the people performing the tasks assured so that the scan operator or the person supervising the scan can be assured of the patient's safety? (For more information on accountability please see the Resources section)	

Table 2.3 Safety Processes to Consider, Post-Screening

Safety Considerations, Post Screening: Scan Room/Zone 4	Factors to Consider	Notes
Protecting hearing	IEC recommend that if equipment is capable of producing more than 99 dB(A), hearing protection should be used. MHRA say 'hearing protection shall always be provided for patients and volunteers unless it can be demonstrated that noise levels will not exceed 80 dB(A)'. If the noise level exceeds this, it's recommended that staff and others in the scan room during a scan wear earplugs and/or ear defenders. The selected hearing protection should be chosen to match the noise frequency spectrum of the MR system and to reduce noise at the eardrum to below 85 dB(A).The scanner manufacturer can be asked to supply information on the maximum noise levels. Earplugs, ear defenders, or other means of hearing protection can be used. Consider how to protect the hearing of those of particular concern such as anaesthetised, incapacitated and paediatric patients and neonates, the fetus and those with pre-existing aural conditions. Neonatal hearing protection can include various types and combinations e.g., soft ear plugs, specially adapted small ear muffs and other specialised aids. If appropriate to do so, consider implementing software options to achieve quieter sequences. Staff should be trained in what hearing protection to select for others and how to properly fit the protection. Do you know what protection the manufacturer's headphones and/or ear plugs provide? Is it recommended that both headphones and ear plugs be worn by patients (and for any staff who may be present in the scan room?). Is there a process to follow if anyone refuses to wear hearing protection?	

(Continued)

Safety Considerations, Post Screening: Scan Room/Zone 4	Factors to Consider	Notes
Example of a typical sign to tell people they are entering an area where hearing is to be protected. 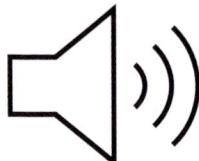	Has a risk assessment been performed, and guidance developed to protect the patient, and those accompanying or supervising the patient for their scan, from excessive noise? Is an appropriate sign on the scan room door warning about the need to wear hearing protection required?	
Communication 	Has the patient's ID been checked as per a standard protocol? Consider what to tell the patient to inform them of what to expect when being scanned. For example, can the patient (and any accompanying person in the scan room) be given an approximate time the scan will take, told to expect a certain kind of noise, and made aware that the table will move etc.? How can it be ensured that the patient knows how to communicate with the scan operator during the scan? Can you, for example, test and show the patient how the patient call system works (buzzer/ squeeze ball/ button) and explain how you will be able to hear them and how they will hear you? Can you check if there is two-way communication with the patient through the intercom before starting the scan? By speaking to the patient at appropriate times during the scan this may highlight any issues early and help to resolve them. What processes can be put in place where adaptations to the routine communication system are required, e.g. for those who cannot squeeze a buzzer, or for deaf or blind patients or those with cognitive impairment? Consider providing written instructions for those with hearing loss to explain beforehand what will be required during the scan. Picture cards and storyboards could be used for young patients and those with learning difficulties. If a patient can't squeeze the buzzer, they could be asked to move their foot, for example, to indicate when they need to communicate. Where breathing instructions are required, pre-agreed physical prompts, such as their foot being touched, could inform a blind or deaf person when to hold their breath.	

Safety Considerations, Post Screening: Scan Room/Zone 4	Factors to Consider	Notes
MR Authorised staff	What MR Authorised staff are permitted entry to the CAA and the scan room and under what circumstances?	
	How can it be ensured that only MR Authorised staff are permitted into the CAA/scan room?	
	Is there a record kept of who the MR Authorised staff are and the type of authorisation they have e.g. which areas they are permitted to enter or to supervise others in etc.? Who is responsible for keeping the list current and making it available?	
	How can you keep entry strictly controlled and ensure only the appropriate MR Authorised staff are permitted to allow others entry into the CAA (i.e. permit only those MR Authorised staff who have been trained in the required screening of others to supervise entry into the CAA etc.).	
	How is MR safety training of all MR Authorised staff maintained?	
	Can auditable safety training be provided on a regular basis?	
Equipment labels Reproduced with permission of the MHRA under the terms of the Open Government Licence (OGL) v3.0	How do you ensure equipment is MR Safe or MR Conditional?	
	Is there an inventory of MR Safe/Conditional equipment?	
	Who is responsible for testing and labelling equipment?	
	How can it be confirmed, where appropriate, that any equipment returned from service or repair is still as expected regarding its MR safety status? For example, how is it ensured that an MR Conditional oxygen cylinder or an MR Conditional fire extinguisher, returned after a refill, still have any expected non ferrous parts? Is there a process to follow for checking and who is responsible for checking? Instructions on the safe process/system for checking any equipment, how to test and label any equipment and what tools to use could be included in a SOP/local guidance.	
	The testing and labelling of items to indicate their MR safety status are described in the ASTM international standard F2503-13. The MHRA recommend having access to a strong (> 0.1 T) handheld magnet or ferromagnetic detector for testing equipment.	

Labelling Items for MR Safety Conditions of Use

The Definitions and Labelling used for Marking Equipment Taken Into the MR Environment

The MHRA recommends testing and labelling of all equipment that will be taken into the MR Environment.

MR SAFE 'an item that poses no known hazards resulting from exposure to any MR environment. MR Safe items are composed of materials that are electrically nonconductive, nonmetallic, and nonmagnetic' *	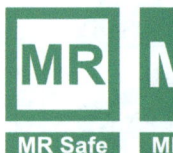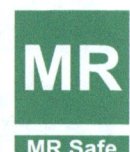
MR CONDITIONAL 'an item with demonstrated safety in the MR environment within defined conditions. At a minimum, address the conditions of the static magnetic field, the switched gradient magnetic field and the radiofrequency fields. Additional conditions, including specific configurations of the item, may be required.'	
MR UNSAFE 'an item which poses unacceptable risks to the patient, medical staff or other persons within the MR environment.'	
MR ENVIRONMENT 'the three dimensional volume of space surrounding the MR magnet that contains both the Faraday shielded volume and the 0.50 mT field contour (5 gauss (G) line). This volume is the region in which an item might pose a hazard from exposure to the electromagnetic fields produced by the MR equipment and accessories.'	

* the updated definition now specifically prohibits items containing conductive, metallic and magnetic materials.

Figure 2.2 Definitions from ASTM International Standard F2503-13 (also published as IEC standard 62570:2014)

Reproduced with permission of the MHRA under the terms of the Open Government Licence (OGL) v3.0

MR Conditions of Use

The MHRA describes how the labelling of MR Conditional should specify information such as:

- Maximum magnetic field in which the device was tested
- Magnitude and location of the maximum spatial gradient
- Maximum rate of change of the gradient field
- RF fields tolerated in terms of RF interference, RF heating and type of transmit mode

Whenever changes are made to the MR Environment, such as a change of scanner field strength, upgrading or replacing the MR system etc., then the safety status of equipment/devices which were previously considered MR Conditional will need to be re-examined.

MR Conditional Labelling to Indicate the Conditions of Use in the MR Environment

Signage below shows the types of labelling used on equipment to indicate the conditions of use in the MR Environment. Where possible, the appropriate descriptive text should be used on labels to describe the conditions.

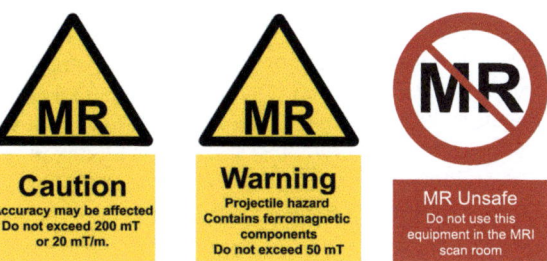

Figure 2.3 Examples of MR Conditional Labelling and an MR Unsafe Label.

Images courtesy of Dr Cormac McGrath, Northern Ireland Regional Medical Physics Service, Belfast Health and Social Care Trust.

The MHRA uses the term MR Unlabelled for items that are not labelled. MR Unlabelled items should be considered to be MR Unsafe until determined to be otherwise. A suggested template for recording unlabelled devices can be seen in Table 2.14.

MR UNLABELLED – an item without any of the following labels:

MR SAFE   MR CONDITIONAL   MR UNSAFE

MRI Department Safety Signage

As well as ensuring that access to the MR CAA is properly controlled, appropriate safety signs should be placed to warn of the risks of entering the area. Good examples of notices that are freely available to download and modify can be found at: https://www.ipem.ac.uk/resources/mri-safety-notices-magnetic-resonance-imaging/ (some are available in various languages).

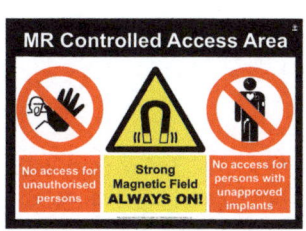
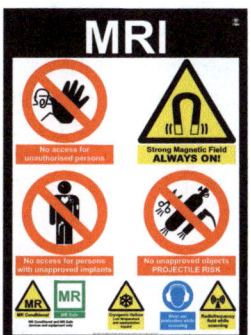

Figure 2.4 Examples of Safety Signage from IPEM.

Notices reproduced courtesy of IPEM.

Considerations to Prevent Patient Burns and Overheating

Table 2.4 Considerations to Prevent Patient Burns and Overheating

If a patient burn occurs, is there a process to follow to ensure immediate treatment is administered? Does the process include reporting the incident as an adverse event or similar, as per the local policy and procedures?

Consideration	Action to Consider	Reason	Notes
Appropriate patient preparation	Could patients be routinely changed out of their own clothes into MR Safe clothing such as pocketless scrubs? Should their underwear be changed too, in case it contains metallic components and is within the area being scanned? How do you know if they are wearing thermal clothing? What checking processes can be put in place to try to ensure that any external metal or other electrically conductive items, deemed necessary to be removed from the patient (hair grips, jewellery, electronic devices etc.) are identified? Could allowing a blanket or sheet overheat the patient? Be aware that a light-weight sheet, if appropriate, may help to maintain patient dignity issues in respect to views down the bore/CCTV monitoring, if the patient is wearing a gown etc. Is there a checking process to find out if hospital linen contains RFID tags?	Wearing MR Safe attire could prevent heating from metallic fibres or treatments in fabric and metallic items (buttons, zips etc.) if pocketless, could avoid heating from forgotten metallic items left in pockets (also prevents a projectile incident, if ferrous). Thermal clothes are designed to maintain or increase body heat. Electrically conductive items can potentially have a current induced if exposed to the EMFs. Unless safe conditions of use can be met or are known, is there guidance to describe when any conductive items are to be removed?	
	Is there a process to follow if the patient is wearing eye make-up and the eyes will be exposed to RF? Consider providing make-up remover products.	Cosmetics (mascara and eye liner) could contain metal particles, which may have the potential to heat up and/ or cause image artefact if exposed to the RF field.	

Consideration	Action to Consider	Reason	Notes
	After removing unrequired metallic or electrically conductive items from the patient, how can you deal with those which cannot be easily removed (e.g. a dermal piercing, tight wedding band, bio-hacking device etc.)?	Metal or electronic items can potentially heat up or be damaged if exposed to the EMFs and can cause image artefact. Is there guidance on how to proceed or to conduct an appropriate risk-versus-benefit analysis?	
	Has the use of FMDs been considered as part of the screening process to identify ferrous metal? If so, is there guidance on how they are to be used?	FMDs may be considered a useful tool for detecting ferrous metal but are only intended to be an adjunct to screening. They are not to be solely relied upon for screening purposes as they are not designed to detect non-ferrous metal, specific implants or all foreign bodies.	
	Is there a process to follow if there are potential concerns of excess water on the patient, such as a wet nappy, or hair etc.?	Water is a conductor.	
Metallic or electrically conductive items in the bore.	Is there a checking process to follow which helps to raise awareness of, and to remove any unused coils, plugs, connectors, cables, wires, devices or any other unrequired conductive items from the bore before scanning the patient?	Prevents patient contact with objects that could potentially heat up (also removes the risk of image artefacts/degradation caused by magnetic field inhomogeneities due to metal in the bore and inhomogenous fat saturation).	

(Continued)

MRI Safety Information

Consideration	Action to Consider	Reason	Notes
Appropriate patient positioning Examples of some do's and dont's to consider when positioning a patient for a typical right shoulder MRI scan in a cylindrical bore. Image courtesy of Johnathan Hewis, Senior Lecturer in Medical Imaging, Charles Sturt University, School of Dentistry and Medical Sciences, Port Macquarie, Australia	Prevent skin-to skin contact and closed, flesh conductive loops from forming through awareness of patient positioning and by incorporating appropriate padding. Is there a process to follow to try to prevent hands from clasping, arms and legs from crossing each other, feet or limbs from touching each other and to try to make sure fingers or finger tips are not touching the patient's body and creating a large conductive flesh loop? The depictions of potential patient positioning seen here are designed to act as reminders to avoid conductive loops from forming and to use appropriate padding but please be guided by the manufacturer on what padding requirements may be required for each particular MR system..	Electric currents can be created in the patient when exposed to EMFs. This energy dissipates in the body as heat. If flesh loops form, these can potentially become conductors for electrical energy. Heat or tingling my be felt where there are points of contact, potentially indicating a thermal effect. However, the sensation may not be recognised as an early indicator of thermal heating by the patient until the damage is done (a skin burn may not become apparent until some time after the scan). Preventing conductive flesh loops from forming can prevent this type of injury (tingling sensations can also indicate PNS). Where large calibre loops form and small points of contact exist, the heating effects may be greater.	
	As required, and as guided by the manufacturer and the particular MR system requirements (e.g the orientation of the system's magnetic field), place appropriate padding, to prevent conductive loops from forming, to create appropriate separation from the RF transmit element and to introduce separation from other conductive items e.g. coils, cables, plugs, monitoring equipment etc. The MHRA recommends using foam pads of 1–2 cm thickness.	Proximity to the bore wall, close to the RF coil transmitter, can lead to heating concerns due to near field effects. Contact with any electrically conductive items can cause heating concerns. Different MR systems may have different padding or separation requirements.	

Consideration	Action to Consider	Reason	Notes
Integrity of all equipment	Is there a way to ensure auditable, regular inspection and maintenance of any equipment or device that may enter the bore or is placed in the MR Environment?	Any broken or damaged equipment, e.g. frayed cables, wires, damaged plugs, etc. may pose an electrical hazard or malfunction due to inappropriate insulation or other physical damage.	
Appropriate positioning of any necessary electrically conductive equipment in the bore	How are you made aware of the recommendations regarding, the MR safety conditions required for safe use of any electrically conductive items and devices on, or connected to, the patient? Is there an agreed checking process with consequent actions to follow?	Understanding and adhering to the MR safety conditions of equipment means that there is an approved safe process to follow to reduce, for example, the risks of burns, prevent the equipment from malfunctioning or causing some other type of adverse event.	
	Understand how to position cables/wires safely. e.g. position them down the centre of the bore (Z-direction, in cylindrical bores), prevent them running close to the bore wall and from crossing one another or passing diagonally across the patient. Prevent coils and loops from forming.	Reduces the risk of heating effects from near field effects and currents being induced from conductive loops.	
	Use appropriate padding to insulate any cables or wires from the patient.	If a conductor touches the patient there is a risk of heating caused by the conductor being exposed to the EMFs.	
Awareness of potential resonant length of conductive items	Where there is a risk that the length of a conductor, for example an implant, could be the appropriate shape and length to cause heating concerns through resonance, a risk assessment by the local MRSE would likely be performed to decide if it poses a risk of resonant heating (determined by the scanner resonant frequency and proportional to the field strength of the scanner).	The 'Resonant/Antenna length' of a conductor varies at different field strengths (and corresponding transmitted Larmor frequencies). Heating due to this effect is related to several factors e.g. length, shape, position, scanner's resonant frequency and what medium the conductor resides in (air versus tissue).	

(Continued)

MRI Safety Information

Consideration	Action to Consider	Reason	Notes
Appropriate patient monitoring	Monitor the patient visually and verbally for any signs of discomfort or distress. Explain beforehand how they can alert you if they feel anything untoward and to use the call system immediately if they feel any pain or discomfort. Communicate regularly throughout the patient's scan. What methods can be used to identify and address concerns relating to patients who are unable to communicate any heating issues, e.g. anaesthetised patients and neonates or those with learning or communication issues?	If the patient is made aware to alert the scan operator of any concerns, then an appropriate and timely safety intervention may be implemented to prevent a potential thermal incident from occurring or getting worse, e.g. by repositioning of patient padding that may have slipped or by stopping the scan. Consider what extra vigilance is possible to ensure those who cannot communicate are properly monitored.	
Appropriate scanner room ambient conditions	Check the scanner user manual to see what the ambient temperature and humidity should be for scanning and know how to change the humidity, temperature settings and air flow. How can you optimise ventilation in the bore for patients? Is there a process to check that the bore fan is working properly? Are there any special heating or cooling considerations required for certain types of patients such as neonates or thermally compromised patients?	Patient heating can be reduced by convection if cool air is circulated through the bore and if room temperature and humidity are appropriate. Following an appropriate risk assessment of the needs of thermally compromised patients, consideration and adjustment of the routine strategies normally used for heating or cooling patients during a scan may be required.	
Awareness of image artefacts	Be aware of image artefacts as indicators of unknown devices or metal. Prompt investigation upon seeing unexpected signal voids, for example, could enable an early intervention to be made. Consider making the initial scout/planning image as large as possible.	Artefacts could represent unknown foreign bodies, electrically conductive materials, metals or coil failures which could cause heating concerns.. An initial large scout/planning image could aid detection of metal in the exposed area, providing an early warning to intervene.	

Consideration	Action to Consider	Reason	Notes
Awareness of tattoos	Tattoos or other types of body art are not considered an explicit contraindication to MRI but may warrant consideration or technique adaptation. Is there guidance to follow? If there are concerns of tattoos heating, what interventions can be made? ACR recommends that a cold compress or ice pack be applied to a tattoo if it's within the volume in which the body coil is being used for RF transmission.. Instruct patients to alert the scan operator immediately if they feel any discomfort, pain or tingling at the site of their tattoo. If the patient has a new tattoo, consider what waiting time (how many hours or days) is appropriate before scanning them. If the patient has reduced or no communication capabilities, consider what adaptations may be required to mitigate the fact that they cannot alert you to any sensations felt.	Tattoos may contain a mixture of chemicals and pigments, and could contain metal/ferromagnetic substances such as iron oxide which is a conductive material, and so may have the potential to heat up if exposed to the transmitted RF.. If the skin has not yet healed from a fresh tattoo, there may be potential for smudging of the fresh design. Early warning by the patient of discomfort or tingling effects alerts the scan operator to potential problems. Appropriate interventions can then be made, such as a cold compress applied to the tattoo site, or stopping the scan to prevent any further potential heating effects or pain sensations.	
Appropriate sequence setup	Understand the meaning of low SAR sequences, scanning in normal mode and why an accurate weight (and height, if required by the system) are factors of SAR management. If scanning in a controlled mode, are the agreed conditions for using this mode, detailed in the local guidance/SOP instructions? (For more information, see Mode of Operation Considerations section).	Certain sequences expose the patient to more energy than others, which is dissipated in the patient as heat. An accurate weight (and height, if required by the system) are factors of SAR management (for more information, see Understanding SAR and B1+rms section).	

MRI Safety Information

Understanding SAR and B1+rms

Internal body heating during MRI is caused by the absorption of electromagnetic power, estimated as the SAR (measured in units of watts per kilogram (W/kg) with time.

SAR is specific to the body part being imaged and is estimated for each sequence by the MRI system software and monitored in real-time by the system hardware. Both peak and time-averaged whole body SAR are reported.

The SAR calculation requires the mass of exposed tissue, usually the patient's weight for convenience, but other models can be used for the head or knee when using dedicated transmit/receive (Tx/Rx) coils, or for low weight patients, e.g., neonates. It is extremely important that an accurate body weight, and height if required, is entered into the MR system.

The average SAR limit is applied over a 6-minute period, whereas a peak SAR of twice the average SAR is allowed over a 10-second period. Heat, or energy, is power (SAR) multiplied by time. If we want to reduce heating, then ideally, we should provide time gaps between sequences.

Please note that SAR increases with the square of the field strength, so the SAR at 3 T will be approximately four times that at 1.5 T for an identical sequence.

The disadvantage of SAR is that it is patient dependent. This makes it very difficult for implant manufacturers to provide accurate SAR limits for their devices, hence they may choose very conservative values.

An alternative way to determine the RF exposure is to use the time average (root mean square or rms) of the RF magnetic field used for excitation, known as B1+rms, which is averaged over a 10-second period. This measurement is based on the actual RF pulses used in the sequence and is determined by MR physics and not the patient. B1+rms is usually measured in units of micro-tesla (µT).

Manufacturers must 'model the SAR', i.e., from the sequence parameters they must estimate how much SAR will get deposited in the body. B1+rms is 'model independent', i.e., the B1+rms should be the same for all scanner types for identical RF pulses and timings.

Some parameters that affect B1+rms are the RF pulse duration and amplitude (which dictates the flip angle) and the number of pulses in a 10-second period (which could be influenced by multi-slice acquisitions/refocusing pulses/fat sat pulses/spatial sat pulses etc.). B1+rms is therefore the recommended scanner output measurement for assessing device safety.

Table 2.5 Typical High and Low SAR Pulse Sequences

Name some of your systems' corresponding specific pulse sequences.

(Please confirm all the latest acronyms and pulse sequences with your vendor as the descriptions below cannot be guaranteed. Cross-vendor terminology can be found at some of the scanner manufacturer's websites as per the Resources section).

Sequence Name	Likely Higher SAR & B1+rms	Likely Lower SAR & B1+rms
	SE	GRE, FISP, FIELD ECHO, FAST FIELD ECHO (FFE), GE
	FSE, TSE	SPGR, FLASH, FAST FE, T1-FFE RSSG
	3D FSE/SE	Magnetisation-prepared Fast Gradient ECHO, BRAVO, MP-RAGE
	STIR	EPI
	FLAIR, Turbo Dark Fluid	SWI, SWAN, FSBB, VENOUS BOLD
	BSSFP, PSIF, T2-FFE, Time Reversed Sarge	
	3D TOF MRA (if with magnetisation transfer preparation)	
	PROPELLER, BLADE, JET, MULTIVANE, RADAR	
	Simultaneous Multi-slice/ Multiband Excitation	

Table 2.6 Considerations to Reduce SAR

For each method to reduce SAR listed in the table below, consider the potential consequences on image quality and/or time.

(For more information on SAR please see the Resources section.)

Considerations to Reduce SAR	Consequences
Modes of operation (use normal vs 1st-level controlled mode)	
Increase repetition time (TR)	
Decrease number of phase encoding steps (use parallel imaging/compressed sensing)	
Reduce excitation flip angles (and, where appropriate, reduce refocusing flip angles)	
Reduce number of slices (keeping TR the same)	
Reduce number of signal averages (NSA, NEX)	
Eliminate pre saturation bands, fat saturation pulses, magnetisation transfer (for 3D TOF MRA)	
Alternate high SAR sequences with low SAR sequences	
Use a lower SAR alternative sequence, e.g. GRE rather than SE	
Reduce the number of echoes (ETL)	
Scan at lower field strengths	
Number of concatenations. Concatenations are a way of equally distributing slices over multiple TRs. Increasing the no. of concatenations allows more slices to fit into a specific TR but increases the TR.	
Introduce pauses between sequences	

Mode of Operation Considerations

The MHRA recommends a three-mode approach to the clinical operation of MRI equipment in line with IEC, HPA & ICNIRP. The information in tables 2.7 – 2.10 is condensed from the MHRA and IEC. For more information, see MHRA Safety Guidelines for MRI Equipment in Clinical Use.

Table 2.7 Summary of Operating Modes

Mode of Operation	Description	Notes
Normal (MHRA)	When risk of ill effect to the patient is minimised.	
Normal (IEC)	Where none of the outputs have a value that may cause physiological stress to patients.	
Controlled (MHRA)	When the exposure is higher than normal mode and the patient will benefit by the enhanced imaging performance. Although the risks are minimised, some people may experience some effects, such as sensory disturbance or transient discomfort due to PNS. Scanning requires patient monitoring.	The MHRA advises that MRI units should develop protocols for the medical supervision and monitoring of patients to be scanned in the controlled mode. In most cases, visual supervision of a conscious patient by the MR Operator will be sufficient to ensure the patient's safety. The number of sequences should be limited to those that are necessary. Pregnant women should not normally be exposed above the lower advised levels of restriction. Protocols should include: • Groups of patients for whom monitoring is appropriate • Parameters to be monitored • Burn prevention • Detail of what parameter changes are significant and what changes are artefacts caused by the static field • Who should be responsible for interpreting the results of any monitoring • How to obtain appropriate medical help when required

(*Continued*)

Mode of Operation	Description	Notes
First level controlled (IEC)	In which one or more outputs reach a value that may cause physiological stress to patients which needs to be controlled by medical supervision.	The IEC recommends medical supervision of patients undergoing scanning in the controlled mode. Medical supervision should include arrangements for the medical management of patients who may be at risk from some parameters of exposure due to their medical condition, the levels of exposure or a combination of both. Requires a positive assessment by a qualified medical practitioner of the risk versus benefit for a particular scan, or a decision by a qualified practitioner that the patient satisfies a set of objective criteria, formulated by a medical practitioner, for the parameters of the scan and the condition of the patient. Medical supervision may entail physiological monitoring.
Research / Experimental (MHRA)	When exposure is only restricted to prevent harmful effects.	Requires approval of a research ethics committee and patient monitoring.
Second level controlled (IEC)	In which one or more outputs reach a value that may produce significant risk for patients.	Explicit ethics committee approval is required.

If operating in First level/Controlled mode, does your local guidance detail when this mode is to be used and under what conditions it should be enabled? If scanning in a controlled mode has a risk-benefit analysis been performed as per the local procedures?. Know how to check what mode you are working in, and how to change the mode and at what point in the scan protocol.

Please always check the latest MHRA guidance to remain current with latest guidance in case new standards are to be adopted.

Static Magnetic Fields

The operating modes below are chosen in respect to potential effects from the **static magnetic fields (B_0):** to prevent effects caused by motion-induced currents caused by B_0. It's recommended that patients are moved slowly into and out of the magnet bore, to avoid the possibility of vertigo and nausea.

Table 2.8 Mode of Operation Considerations: Static Magnetic Fields (B_0)

Operating Mode	Consequences of Restrictions to Reduce Potential Effects from Static Magnetic Fields (B_0)
Normal	Patient should not experience effects such as vertigo, dizziness or nausea
Controlled	Some patients may experience effects such as vertigo, dizziness or nausea
Research/Experimental	Exposure is unrestricted

Time-varying Magnetic Field Gradients

The modes below are chosen in respect to potential effects from **time-varying magnetic field gradients (dB/dt):** to restrict PNS and to prevent cardiac muscle stimulation.

Table 2.9 Mode of Operation Considerations: Time-varying Magnetic Field Gradients (dB/dt)

Operating Mode	Consequences of Restrictions to Reduce Potential Effects from Time-varying Magnetic Field Gradients (dB/dt)
Normal	The gradient system shall operate at a level that does not exceed 80% of the mean threshold for PNS, where the threshold for PNS is defined as the onset of sensation (IEC/ICNIRP/HPA) Some patients may experience PNS but uncomfortable PNS is prevented (MHRA)
Controlled	The gradient system shall operate at a level that does not exceed 100% of the directly determined mean threshold for PNS (first level controlled, IEC/ICNIRP/HPA) Some patients may experience uncomfortable PNS (MHRA)
Research/Experimental	ICNIRP has no limit for experimental mode exposures, IEC has a limit to prevent cardiac stimulation and HPA has suggested that a limit of 120% of the directly determined mean threshold for PNS. Exposure is restricted to prevent cardiac stimulation (MHRA).

RF Magnetic Fields (B_1)

The modes below are chosen with respect to potential effects from **RF magnetic fields (B_1):** to restrict SAR such that temperature rise is restricted. The basic restriction is to limit whole body temperature rise under moderate environmental conditions.

Table 2.10 RF Magnetic Fields (B_1)

Operating Mode	Consequences of Restrictions to Reduce Potential Effects from RF Magnetic Fields (B_1)
Normal	A whole-body temperature rise of >0.5°C will be prevented
Controlled	A whole-body temperature rise of >1°C will be prevented
Research/Experimental	Exposure is restricted in order to avoid tissue damage (<2°C recommended by HPA)

Weight and Height Measurement Conversion Charts

Weight Measurement Conversion Chart

Kilograms	Stones (st) & Pounds (lb)	Pounds	Kilograms	Stones (st) & Pounds (lb)	Pounds
1	2 lbs	2.20	135	21 st 4 lbs	297.62
5	11 lbs	11.02	140	22 st 1 lbs	308.65
10	1 st 8 lbs	22.05	145	22 st 12 lbs	319.67
15	2 st 5 lbs	33.07	150	23 st 9 lbs	330.69
20	3 st 2 lbs	44.09	155	24 st 6 lbs	341.72
25	3 st 13 lbs	55.12	160	25 st 3 lbs	352.74
30	4 st 10 lbs	66.14	165	26 st 0 lbs	363.76
35	5 st 7 lbs	77.16	170	26 st 11 lbs	374.79
40	6 st 4 lbs	88.18	175	27 st 8 lbs	385.81
45	7 st 1 lbs	99.21	180	28 st 5 lbs	396.83
50	7 st 12 lbs	110.23	185	29 st 2 lbs	407.85
55	8 st 9 lbs	121.25	190	29 st 13 lbs	418.88
60	9 st 6 lbs	132.28	195	30 st 10 lbs	429.90
65	10 st 3 lbs	143.30	200	31 st 7 lbs	440.92
70	11 st 0 lbs	154.32	205	32 st 4 lbs	451.95
75	11 st 11 lbs	165.35	210	33 st 1 lbs	462.97
80	12 st 8 lbs	176.37	215	33 st 12 lbs	473.99
85	13 st 5 lbs	187.39	220	34 st 9 lbs	485.02
90	14 st 2 lbs	198.42	225	35 st 6 lbs	496.04
95	14 st 13 lbs	209.44	230	36 st 3 lbs	507.06
100	15 st 10 lbs	220.46	235	37 st 0 lbs	518.09
105	16 st 7 lbs	231.49	240	37 st 11 lbs	529.11
110	17 st 5 lbs	242.51	245	38 st 8 lbs	540.13
115	18 st 2 lbs	253.53	250	39 st 5 lbs	551.16
120	18 st 13 lbs	264.55			
125	19 st 10 lbs	275.58			
130	20 st 7 lbs	286.60			

Height Measurement Conversion Chart

Height			Height		
Centimetres	Metres	Feet and Inches	Centimetres	Metres	Feet and Inches
20	0.2	0' 8"	140	1.4	4' 7"
25	0.25	0' 10"	145	1.45	4' 9"
30	0.3	0' 12"	150	1.5	4' 11"
35	0.35	1' 2"	155	1.55	5' 1"
40	0.4	1' 4"	160	1.6	5' 3"
45	0.45	1' 6"	165	1.65	5' 5"
50	0.5	1' 8"	170	1.7	5' 7"
55	0.55	1' 10"	175	1.75	5' 9"
60	0.6	1' 12"	180	1.8	5' 11"
65	0.65	2' 2"	185	1.85	6' 1"
70	0.7	2' 4"	190	1.9	6' 3"
75	0.75	2' 6"	195	1.95	6' 5"
80	0.8	2' 7"	200	2	6' 7"
85	0.85	2' 9"	205	2.05	6' 9"
90	0.9	2' 11"	210	2.1	6' 11"
95	0.95	3' 1"	215	2.15	7' 1"
100	1	3' 3"	220	2.2	7' 3"
105	1.05	3' 5"	225	2.25	7' 5"
110	1.1	3' 7"	230	2.3	7' 7"
115	1.15	3' 9"			
120	1.2	3' 11"			
125	1.25	4' 1"			
130	1.3	4' 3"			
135	1.35	4' 5"			

Considerations for Managing Implants

Table 2.11 Passive and Active Implant Descriptions

Type of Device or Implant	Description	Examples	Potential Effects (under certain circumstances) on a Device/Implant if Exposed to the EMFs	Notes and where Local Process/Guidance is Located
Passive/ non-active	Devices/implants that require **no power source** to function.	Joint replacements, heart valves, aneurysm clips, stents, abandoned / retained leads etc.	Potential heating, movement and conduction.	
Active	Devices/Implants **which do require an energy source to function** such as electrical, radio wave/ Wi-Fi, mechanical or pneumatic power.	Pacemakers, defibrillators, loop recorders, neurostimulators, cochlear implants, drug pumps, glucose monitoring devices and magnetically activated orthopaedic/growth rod type devices.	Potential heating, movement, conduction, damage and incorrect function of the device.	

A link to information on the development of GISP can be found in the Resources section.

Stages of a Typical MRI Appointment

Referral made
Key questions regarding MRI contraindications would normally be completed by the referring clinician.

Referral received
An administrator will likely enter the referral on the booking system, checking that the referral is signed and the correct patient ID is matched up to the referral. They then add the referral to the correct MRI examination list for vetting (e.g. brain on to a neuro pending list etc.).

Vetting
Guidelines for referral acceptance to be followed. Referral double-checked to ensure nothing is overlooked. Patient details must match criteria for checking and the referral must be justified. Reviewing previous imaging may be required to ensure request is appropriate and not duplicated. Any implant or other concerns can be identified from the questions that the referrer has completed. This stage would ideally also identify if the patient requires additional assistance, e.g., a hoist to lift them onto MR Conditional transport or a translator to be booked for their appointment.

Reviewing relevant previous patient information
If a concern is suspected or identified then review any relevant imaging, reports or warnings on the patient's record to provide further information. Follow the local SOP to investigate any concern. (see Stages of a Typical Implant/FB Investigation for some points to consider).

Pre-appointment screening
If the booking team make the appointment with the patient by phone or if the patient is asked to confirm their appointment by phone, the patient could be asked some key MRI safety questions at this stage. This could prevent a wasted slot or clinical time on the patient's appointment day.

Questionnaire sent in advance
The patient is sent a copy of the safety questionnaire along with their appointment letter and information about their scan in advance of their appointment. Having appropriate contact details included in the paperwork so that the patient may contact the appropriate team to ask any queries or state any concerns could help to identify that there is an unknown implant. It could also enable more time to be scheduled for the patient's appointment if they are anxious, etc.

1st verbal / visual screening
On appointment day, the safety questionnaire and ID are checked with the patient before starting any preparation (as per local protocol). This first check might be done by a support worker, Assistant Practitioner, or Radiographer, trained in MRI safety, as per the local policy.

2nd verbal / visual screening / final checks
After patient screening and patient preparation, final checks are performed such as, the patient's ID and safety screening form, that the referral clinical details match the area being scanned (and the patient's expectations of what part of their body is to be scanned). Pause to double-check anything on, or associated with, the patient before entering the scan room with the patient. These final checks are performed by a suitably MR Authorised person e.g. a Radiographer, the MR Supervisor, MR Responsible Person or Scan Operator, as per the locally agreed process.

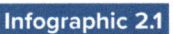 Stages of a Typical MRI Appointment.

MRI Safety Information

Who is authorised to investigate?

At some stage in the MRI safety referral/screening process, a potential unknown implant, surgery or FB may be suspected. The steps below are designed to provide some points to consider when investigating.

Is there a local process to follow and does it, for example, state who has the appropriate authority to follow all the steps in the process to investigate implants etc. and to proceed to scan or not?

Question the patient

Explain why the investigation is required asking what do they know/remember? If inappropriate to ask the patient (non cognitive), but required, is there consent to speak to a family member to try to find out more? Does the local policy permit checking the patient's body for any signs of previous surgery?

Review previous imaging

Is recent previous imaging available? Are hospital notes and/or GP information available? Imaging may indicate if it's a FB or a passive or active implant. Imaging may also reveal its position, shape, size and whether it's likely to be metal.

Implant cards

Does the patient have an implant card / any record of the surgery?

Hospital records

What further imaging is permitted, if required (e.g. X-Rays), to try to identify an implant or FB? If confirmed there is an implant, can you access or request the operation notes and traceability records that will identify the make and model of the implant? Can you contact the referrer or implanting surgeon for more information?

As per local policy, check the MRI safety information related to the implant

If the implant cannot be scanned under a local policy or procedure without further information, can you contact the implant manufacturer direct or access their latest website advice to find out more? Is the implant considered MR Safe, MR Conditional, MR Unsafe or is it MR Unlabelled? If it's MR Conditional, does your system hardware and software allow you to comply with the conditions for scanning the implant?

Still unsure? Check with an appropriate lead

According to your local guidance, who can you turn to for further advice? Is there an MRSE, MR Responsible Person, MRSO or a Radiologist to consult with?

If unsure how to proceed, always seek advice from someone with more experience and knowledge.

Proceed with the scan only when you are satisfied it is safe to do so, in line with your local procedures and policies.

Don't feel pressurised into scanning a patient who has, or may have, an implant or FB if you're not sure how to safely scan the patient or unsure if they should be scanned. Seek guidance from your organisation.

Document the outcome

If the patient is to be scanned, has all appropriate documentation been recorded and signed as required e,g, patient consent, risk assessments, implant forms etc.? Has the patient been informed of the potential risks or outcome for scanning their implant, e.g., reduced image quality? As per the local process, who has the final authority to sign off on the conditions for scanning or on the decision to scan or not? Are there any post-scan procedures to be performed e.g.,organising a programmable shunt or pump to be re-set etc?

What documentation is required if the patient cannot be scanned?

Infographic 2.2 Stages of a Typical Implant or FB Investigation.

Note: The steps above may only be considered if the implant cannot be scanned under a local policy/procedure without further information.
Source: Examples of a Typical MRI Appointment and a Typical Implant or FB Investigation, template design ©yadirainza via Canva.com

Table 2.12 Template for Logging the Procedures for Dealing with Passive Implants

Passive Implant/Device	Name/Type	MR Safe	MR Conditional	MR Unsafe	MR Unlabelled	Notes and where Procedure or Policy and any Reference Material are found
Aneurysm clip						
Annuloplasty ring						
Stents (coronary, peripheral vessel, biliary etc.)						
Dental implant						
External fixation device						
Gastric band						
Heart valves						
Inner ear implant						
IUDs						
IVC filter						
Joint replacement						
Occlusive clips/staples						
Ocular implant						
Sternal wires						
Abandoned/retained wires or leads						

MRI Safety Information

Table 2.13 Template for Logging the Procedures for Dealing with Active Implants

Active Implant/ Device	Name/Type	MR Safe	MR Conditional	MR Unsafe	MR Unlabelled	Notes and where Procedure or Policy and any Reference Material are found
Bio hacking device						
Capsule endoscopy (pill camera)						
CIED						
Cochlear implant						
CGM						
Growth rods (magnetic type)						
Loop recorder						
Medicine Pump						
Neurostimulator						
Programmable shunt						

Unlabelled Devices/Implants

MR Unlabelled describes implants/devices that have not been tested in the MR Environment and are to be considered MR Unsafe until a suitable risk assessment is performed.

Table 2.14 Template for Logging the Procedures for Dealing with Unlabelled Devices/Implants

Unlabelled Implant/ Device Name	Procedure for Investigating	MR Safe	MR Conditional	MR Unsafe	Procedure for Clearance/Sign-off or Refusal	Notes and where Procedure or Policy and any Reference Material are found

Notes

Procedure for Dealing with Unlabelled Devices/Implants

The MHRA describes a process for scanning patients with implants where MRI may be contraindicated but the benefit to the patient outweighs the potential risk of the procedure. It describes the need to follow a careful risk assessment and documentation process, gathering advice and evidence from many sources, undertaken with the full involvement of a multidisciplinary team. The team includes the MR Responsible Person, MRSE, a radiologist (where available), a relevant specialist clinician and the referring clinician. Appropriate precautions are identified and implemented to minimize the risk. Patient consent should be obtained for this procedure. The guidance also advises that an MR unit should not feel under pressure to scan a patient with an unlabelled implant if they do not feel confident to do so. In such circumstances it may be appropriate to refer the patient to another MRI department which has the necessary experience in either scanning that particular device/implant or are more confident in the general application of the scanning procedure required.

Examples of situations where it might be considered necessary to be able to perform an MRI scan on a patient with a device or implant, but MRI is contraindicated, are:

- Where the device or implant is MR Conditional, but the manufacturer's guidance cannot be met
- Where the device or implant is MR Unlabelled or the conditions for scanning it are unknown
- Where the device or implant is known to be MR Unsafe

The risk assessment on the decision as to whether to scan an MR Unlabelled device or implant may include:

- Consideration of using alternative imaging modalities
- Scanning the patient using a scanner with a different field strength and/or gradient fields. This may require referral to a different MRI unit.
- Latest advice from the implant manufacturer
- Assessment of any appropriate Professional Body recommendations regarding the device or implant
- Published evidence of scanning the device
- Provision of procedures to ensure that a suitable clinician is available and in the department at the time of the scan, e.g. for cardiac devices, a cardiologist or cardiac physiologist
- Assessment of possible artefacts
- What data is available about the device, such as:
    - Identification of MRI device parameters and how they may be adjusted to implement appropriate precautions to minimize the risk
    - Appropriate programming of the device
    - Suitable patient monitoring (e.g. SAR levels, physiological signals) during the scan and an appreciation that physiological monitoring may require appropriately trained personnel to operate the monitoring and/or interpret any results
    - SAR exposure considerations including the methods to reduce it, e.g. use of transmit/receive coils (for other methods to reduce SAR, see table 2.6)
- Procedures for post-scan evaluation of the patient.

Table 2.15 Template to Record Implant/Device Information

Implant/Device			
Maximum Magnetic Field Strength that the Implant/Device was Tested at	SAR/B1+rms Values/Limits	Coil Type: Tx/Rx or Rx only	Coil Placement in Relation to Implant/Device
Device Placement/Orientation in Relation to B_0		Slew Rate	
		Max. Spatial Gradient	
Additional Manufacturer Advice, Conditions and Restrictions		Expected Artefact	
		Implant Safety Status	
Pre or Post Scan Instructions/Notes		Implant/Device Location	

Table 2.15 Template to Record Implant/Device Information

Implant/Device			
Maximum Magnetic Field Strength that the Implant/Device was Tested at	**SAR/B1+rms Values/Limits**	**Coil Type: Tx/Rx or Rx only**	**Coil Placement in Relation to Implant/Device**

Device Placement/Orientation in Relation to B_0	Slew Rate
	Max. Spatial Gradient
Additional Manufacturer Advice, Conditions and Restrictions	**Expected Artefact**
	Implant Safety Status
Pre or Post Scan Instructions/Notes	**Implant/Device Location**

Table 2.15 Template to Record Implant/Device Information

Implant/Device			
Maximum Magnetic Field Strength that the Implant/Device was Tested at	SAR/B1+rms Values/Limits	Coil Type: Tx/Rx or Rx only	Coil Placement in Relation to Implant/Device
Device Placement/Orientation in Relation to B_0		Slew Rate	
		Max. Spatial Gradient	
Additional Manufacturer Advice, Conditions and Restrictions		Expected Artefact	
		Implant Safety Status	
Pre or Post Scan Instructions/Notes		Implant/Device Location	

Table 2.15 Template to Record Implant/Device Information

Implant/Device			
Maximum Magnetic Field Strength that the Implant/Device was Tested at	**SAR/B1+rms Values/Limits**	**Coil Type: Tx/Rx or Rx only**	**Coil Placement in Relation to Implant/Device**
Device Placement/Orientation in Relation to B_0		**Slew Rate**	
		Max. Spatial Gradient	
Additional Manufacturer Advice, Conditions and Restrictions		**Expected Artefact**	
		Implant Safety Status	
Pre or Post Scan Instructions/Notes		**Implant/Device Location**	

Table 2.15 Template to Record Implant/Device Information

Implant/Device			
Maximum Magnetic Field Strength that the Implant/Device was Tested at	SAR/B1+rms Values/Limits	Coil Type: Tx/Rx or Rx only	Coil Placement in Relation to Implant/Device
Device Placement/Orientation in Relation to B_0		Slew Rate	
		Max. Spatial Gradient	
Additional Manufacturer Advice, Conditions and Restrictions		Expected Artefact	
		Implant Safety Status	
Pre or Post Scan Instructions/Notes		Implant/Device Location	

Table 2.15 Template to Record Implant/Device Information

Implant/Device			
Maximum Magnetic Field Strength that the Implant/Device was Tested at	SAR/B1+rms Values/Limits	Coil Type: Tx/Rx or Rx only	Coil Placement in Relation to Implant/Device

Device Placement/Orientation in Relation to B_0	Slew Rate
	Max. Spatial Gradient
Additional Manufacturer Advice, Conditions and Restrictions	Expected Artefact
	Implant Safety Status
Pre or Post Scan Instructions/Notes	Implant/Device Location

Notes

3 Equipment Information

Table 3.1 Some Suggested Regular and Planned Checks to Consider

Checks to Consider, in Accordance with your Local Recommendations and Manufacturer's Guidance (Frequency as agreed locally, e.g. daily, weekly, monthly, planned date, etc.)	Frequency of Check	Reading/ Working?
General Checks		
Quality assurance/quality control checks		
Patient table (movement up/down and in/out, docking/undocking, docking table brakes, table emergency release, etc.)		
Oxygen monitor		
MR system helium levels (if possible)		
Chiller		
Sufficient daily stock, e.g. ear plugs, headphone covers, contrast, syringes, gloves, etc.		
Anaesthetic machine and monitor (if trained to do so)		
Contrast injector and pump batteries are fully charged		
Chilled water temperature check		
Visual check of MR equipment room for any water leaks or any other unexpected hazards		
Gas scavenger (if anaesthetic cases)		
Relevant piped medical airflow meters and connections (if trained to do so)		
Image archiving system		
Telephones		
Laser/Landmarking lights		
Patient's entertainment system		

(*Continued*)

Equipment Information

Checks to Consider, in Accordance with your Local Recommendations and Manufacturer's Guidance (Frequency as agreed locally, e.g. daily, weekly, monthly, planned date, etc.)	Frequency of Check	Reading/ Working?
Coils, cables and plugs		
Foam inserts in coils, table pads, positioning aides etc. (checking for cracks etc.)		
Scanning Room Ambient Conditions		
Temperature		
Humidity		
Lighting		
Bore fan operation (working)		
Air Conditioning		
Ventilation		
Emergency/Resuscitation Equipment		
Emergency MR Conditional patient retrieval transport (trolley, wheelchair)		
Oxygen tank (be aware if MR Conditional or MR Unsafe)		
Oxygen masks		
Oxygen flow meter and connections (if on wall)		
Emergency 'Grab bag' or emergency equipment or drugs cart		
Defibrillator		

Checks to Consider, in Accordance with your Local Recommendations and Manufacturer's Guidance (Frequency as agreed locally, e.g. daily, weekly, monthly, planned date, etc.)	Frequency of Check	Reading/ Working?
Portable suction (be aware if MR Conditional or MR Unsafe)		
Suction connection (if on wall)		
Resus trolley/crash cart		
Fire extinguisher		
Fire alarm testing system (if available)		
QA phantom spillage kit		
Medical emergency call systems working		
Patient lift working and any environmental safety concerns (for mobile scanners)		
Anaphylaxis box/drugs		
Patient Call Systems and Monitoring Equipment		
Patient call button/buzzer		
Headphones for patient or anyone in the scan room present during a scan		
CCTV working properly		
Intercom working properly		

(Continued)

Equipment Information

Equipment Information

Checks to Consider, in Accordance with your Local Recommendations and Manufacturer's Guidance (Frequency as agreed locally, e.g. daily, weekly, monthly, planned date, etc.)	Frequency of Check	Reading/ Working?
MR CAA/Scan Room Door(s)		
Check controlled access area doors are locking correctly		
Check RF cage integrity of the scan room door by checking the copper or aluminium RF fingers		
Clean the RF footplate of the scan room cabin door frame to ensure no RF interference occurs because of poor electrical contact between the copper or aluminium RF fingers and the door frame/footplate.		
Check RF doorhandle and escape hatch (if present) are working		
Other Checks		
Quench pipe (by trained specialists)		
Scan room exhaust fan system (by trained specialists)		

Checks to Consider, in Accordance with your Local Recommendations and Manufacturer's Guidance (Frequency as agreed locally, e.g. daily, weekly, monthly, planned date, etc.)	Frequency of Check	Reading/ Working?
Planned Service Dates for Specific Equipment		

Table 3.2 Considerations when Scanning QA/QC Phantom(s)

Process	When to Perform QA, e.g. Daily and as Required Following Appropriate Imaging/Coil Issues	Scan set-up/ Preparation	Scans/ Sequences to Perform	Post Processing	Notes
QA/QC Phantom Scanning Procedure					

Table 3.3 Post-Scanning Considerations: QA/QC Phantom(s)

Process	Desired Results	Passed/ Failed	Escalation Policy if Failed	Where Results are to be Recorded	Recorded By	Notes
Post Scan QA/QC Phantom Procedure						

Equipment Information

Table 3.4 Template for Recording Specific Scanner Information

Equipment Information			
Location/Site:		Field Strength:	
Vendor/Manufacturer:		Type (Superconductive, Resistive, Permanent, Cylindrical, Open Bore, Closed Bore, Upright, etc.):	
System Username:		Magnetic Field Orientation:	
Software Version: Date of Installation:		Max Slew Rate (T/m/s):	
Application Entity Title (AET):		Max Spatial Gradient (T/m or G/cm):	
IP Address/DICOM Port:			
Bore Diameter Size:		Static Field (B_0): 1 T = 10,000 G	
Bore Vertical Size Limit:		B_0 Spatial Field Gradient (SFG): 1 T/m = 100 G/cm	
Bore Horizontal Size Limit:		Imaging Gradients: 10 mT/m = 1 G/cm	
Table Weight Limit:		RF field (B_1): 1 µT = 10 G	
Cylindrical Bore Measurements	**Alternative Shaped Bore Measurements**	Room Temperature:	
		Room Humidity:	
		Repair and Maintenance Contract:	
		Chilled Water Temperature:	
		Flow Rate:	
Contour Plot/Map of Spatial Gradient, Highlighting Maximum Spatial Gradient		Table Emergency Extract Mechanism Location:	
		Coil/Serial No.	Tx/Rx or Rx

Table 3.4 Template for Recording Specific Scanner Information

Location/Site:		Field Strength:	
Vendor/Manufacturer:		Type (Superconductive, Resistive, Permanent, Cylindrical, Open Bore, Closed Bore, Upright etc.):	
System Username:		Magnetic Field Orientation:	
Software Version:	Date of Installation:	Max Slew Rate (T/m/s):	
Application Entity Title (AET):		Max Spatial Gradient (T/m or G/cm):	
IP Address/DICOM Port:			
Bore Diameter Size:		Static Field (B_0): 1 T = 10,000 G	
Bore Vertical Size Limit:		B_0 Spatial Field Gradient (SFG): 1 T/m = 100 G/cm	
Bore Horizontal Size Limit:		Imaging Gradients: 10 mT/m = 1 G/cm	
Table Weight Limit:		RF field (B_1): 1 µT = 10 G	
Cylindrical Bore Measurements	**Alternative Shaped Bore Measurements**	Room Temperature:	
		Room Humidity:	
		Repair and Maintenance Contract:	
		Chilled Water Temperature:	
		Flow Rate:	
Contour Plot/Map of Spatial Gradient, Highlighting Maximum Spatial Gradient		Table Emergency Extract Mechanism Location:	
		Coil/Serial No.	**Tx/Rx or Rx**

Equipment Information

Table 3.4 Template for Recording Specific Scanner Information

Equipment Information			
Location/Site:		Field Strength:	
Vendor/Manufacturer:		Type (Superconductive, Resistive, Permanent, Cylindrical, Open Bore, Closed Bore, Upright etc.):	
System Username:		Magnetic Field Orientation:	
Software Version: Date of Installation:		Max Slew Rate (T/m/s):	
Application Entity Title (AET):		Max Spatial Gradient (T/m or G/cm):	
IP Address/DICOM Port:			
Bore Diameter Size:		Static Field (B_0): 1 T = 10,000 G	
Bore Vertical Size Limit:		B_0 Spatial Field Gradient (SFG): 1 T/m = 100 G/cm	
Bore Horizontal Size Limit:		Imaging Gradients: 10 mT/m = 1 G/cm	
Table Weight Limit:		RF field (B_1): 1 µT = 10 G	
Cylindrical Bore Measurements	Alternative Shaped Bore Measurements	Room Temperature:	
		Room Humidity:	
		Repair and Maintenance Contract:	
		Chilled Water Temperature:	
		Flow Rate:	
Contour Plot/Map of Spatial Gradient, Highlighting Maximum Spatial Gradient		Table Emergency Extract Mechanism Location:	
		Coil/Serial No.	Tx/Rx or Rx

Table 3.4 Template for Recording Specific Scanner Information

Location/Site:		**Field Strength:**
Vendor/Manufacturer:		**Type (Superconductive, Resistive, Permanent, Cylindrical, Open Bore, Closed Bore, Upright etc.):**
System Username:		**Magnetic Field Orientation:**
Software Version:	Date of Installation:	**Max Slew Rate (T/m/s):**
Application Entity Title (AET):		**Max Spatial Gradient (T/m or G/cm):**
IP Address/DICOM Port:		
Bore Diameter Size:		**Static Field (B_0): 1 T = 10,000 G**
Bore Vertical Size Limit:		**B_0 Spatial Field Gradient (SFG): 1 T/m = 100 G/cm**
Bore Horizontal Size Limit:		**Imaging Gradients: 10 mT/m = 1 G/cm**
Table Weight Limit:		**RF field (B_1): 1 µT = 10 G**
Cylindrical Bore Measurements	**Alternative Shaped Bore Measurements**	Room Temperature:
		Room Humidity:
		Repair and Maintenance Contract:
		Chilled Water Temperature:
		Flow Rate:
Contour Plot/Map of Spatial Gradient, Highlighting Maximum Spatial Gradient		Table Emergency Extract Mechanism Location:
		Coil/Serial No. | Tx/Rx or Rx

Table 3.4 Template for Recording Specific Scanner Information

Location/Site:		Field Strength:	
Vendor/Manufacturer:		Type (Superconductive, Resistive, Permanent, Cylindrical, Open Bore, Closed Bore, Upright etc.):	
System Username:		Magnetic Field Orientation:	
Software Version:	Date of Installation:	Max Slew Rate (T/m/s):	
Application Entity Title (AET):		Max Spatial Gradient (T/m or G/cm):	
IP Address/DICOM Port:			
Bore Diameter Size:		Static Field (B_0): 1 T = 10,000 G	
Bore Vertical Size Limit:		B_0 Spatial Field Gradient (SFG): 1 T/m = 100 G/cm	
Bore Horizontal Size Limit:		Imaging Gradients: 10 mT/m = 1 G/cm	
Table Weight Limit:		RF field (B_1): 1 µT = 10 G	
Cylindrical Bore Measurements	Alternative Shaped Bore Measurements	Room Temperature:	
		Room Humidity:	
		Repair and Maintenance Contract:	
		Chilled Water Temperature:	
		Flow Rate:	
Contour Plot/Map of Spatial Gradient, Highlighting Maximum Spatial Gradient		Table Emergency Extract Mechanism Location:	
		Coil/Serial No.	Tx/Rx or Rx

Equipment Information

Table 3.4 Template for Recording Specific Scanner Information

Location/Site:		Field Strength:
Vendor/Manufacturer:		Type (Superconductive, Resistive, Permanent, Cylindrical, Open Bore, Closed Bore, Upright etc.):
System Username:		Magnetic Field Orientation:
Software Version:	Date of Installation:	Max Slew Rate (T/m/s):
Application Entity Title (AET):		Max Spatial Gradient (T/m or G/cm):
IP Address/DICOM Port:		
Bore Diameter Size:		Static Field (B_0): 1 T = 10,000 G
Bore Vertical Size Limit:		B_0 Spatial Field Gradient (SFG): 1 T/m = 100 G/cm
Bore Horizontal Size Limit:		Imaging Gradients: 10 mT/m = 1 G/cm
Table Weight Limit:		RF field (B_1): 1 µT = 10 G
Cylindrical Bore Measurements	**Alternative Shaped Bore Measurements**	Room Temperature:
		Room Humidity:
		Repair and Maintenance Contract:
		Chilled Water Temperature:
		Flow Rate:
Contour Plot/Map of Spatial Gradient, Highlighting Maximum Spatial Gradient		Table Emergency Extract Mechanism Location:
		Coil/Serial No.	Tx/Rx or Rx

Equipment Information

Table 3.5 A Typical Equipment Repair and Maintenance Records Template

Suggested Content to Include for Equipment Repair and Maintenance Records
Fault:
Date:
Process for cancelling or re-booking patients:
Save log/system record of fault/issue:
Equipment:
Date Manufacturer/Vendor/Customer Service Informed:
Job Reference Number:
Date Resolved:
Downtime:
Results of Downtime:
Process for Taking Equipment Out of Service/Decommission:
Reporter:
Example of an Equipment Handover form, to be supplied to the service engineer or maintenance/customer service personnel upon return of any equipment for use, is available from AXREM to download at: https://www.axrem.org.uk/resource/general-equipment-handover-form/

Equipment Information

Table 3.6 Names and Types of Coils

Transmit and Receive (Tx/Rx)	Receive Only (Rx)	Coil Positioning/Notes

Coil Type

MRI coils are offered in a variety of shapes and sizes, designed to accommodate specific body parts.

All coils should be clearly labelled as Transmit and Receive, or Receive only.

1. Transmit and Receive: Tx/Rx
2. Receive only: Rx

Tx/Rx coils are usually identifiable by the presence of a transmit pin in the plug. They should only be connectable to a dedicated Tx/Rx port, that can support both transmit and receive. As far as the author is aware, at the time of writing, there are no detachable transmit coils commercially available.

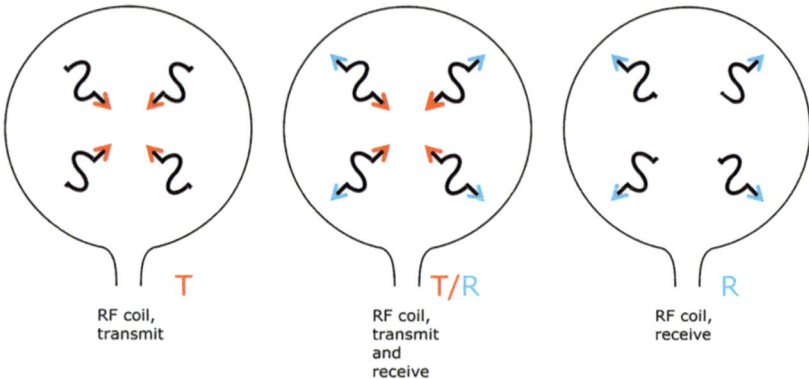

Compliant coil labelling from IEC 60601-2-33
(arrow heads may be in black and white and not colour).

Infographic 3.1 Compliant Coil Labelling.

Image created and supplied courtesy of Professor Martin J. Graves, Professor of MR Physics, University of Cambridge.

Safety conditions for some implanted devices will specify the type of coil that may be used for a specific MRI examination.

Notes

Notes

4 Pulse Sequence Information and Considerations

Table 4.1 Template for Recording Pulse Sequence Parameters and Information

Protocol Name or No.	Field Strength	FOV (PE × FE) [x SE for 3D] (cm)	Matrix (PE × FE) [x SE for 3D]	SL/Gap (mm or %)	TR (ms)	TE (ms)	TI (ms)	ETL/ TF	RBW (±kHz) or (Hz/pixel) or WFS (pixel)	Flip (°)	Other Information, e.g., Imaging Options, FatSat, SpSat, Contrast Agent, Coil, etc.

PE = Phase encoding; FE = Frequency encoding; SE = (Slice encoding – for 3D); SL = Slice thickness; TR= Repetition time; TE = Echo time; TI = Inversion Time; ETL = Echo train length; TF = Turbo factor; RBW = Receiver bandwidth; WFS = Water Fat Shift; Flip = Excitation or refocusing flip angle.

Pulse Sequence Information and Considerations

Table 4.1a Template for Recording Protocol Information

Protocol Name or No.	Body Area	Clinical Indication	Variants	Notes

Table 4.2 Template for Noting Scanner Manufacturers' Pulse Sequence Terminology

The manufacturers below are placed in alphabetical order. For manufacturers' websites and links to cross-vendor pulse sequence terminology, please see the Resources section.

Canon Medical	Esaote	Fujifilm	General Electric (GE)	Philips	Siemens	United Imaging Healthcare

Pulse Sequence Information and Considerations

Table 4.3 Pulse Sequence Parameter Trade-Offs

Parameter	Action	Signal to Noise Ratio	Spatial Resolution	Time	T1 Weighting	T2 Weighting	PD Weighting	Notes
TR	INCREASE	INCREASE	X	INCREASE	DECREASE	INCREASE	INCREASE	
TE	INCREASE	DECREASE	X	X	DECREASE	INCREASE	DECREASE	
FOV	INCREASE	INCREASE	DECREASE	X	X	X	X	
Frequency Matrix	INCREASE	DECREASE	INCREASE	X	X	X	X	
Phase Matrix	INCREASE	DECREASE	INCREASE	INCREASE	X	X	X	
RBW/ Bandwidth	INCREASE	DECREASE	X	X	X	X	X	
NEX/Averages/ NSA	INCREASE	INCREASE	X	INCREASE	X	X	X	
Slice Thickness	INCREASE	INCREASE	DECREASE	X	X	X	X	
ETL FSE/ETL	INCREASE	DECREASE	DECREASE	DECREASE	X	X	X	
Refocusing Flip Angle (FSE/TSE)	DECREASE	DECREASE	X	X	INCREASE	X	X	

Table 4.4 General Considerations When Planning Slices and Sequences

Consideration	Information/Actions to Consider
Direction of Slices	Typically: 　Superior to inferior 　Right to left 　Anterior to posterior Some manufacturers coordinate slice direction differently e.g., Posterior to Anterior. Understand their anatomical labelling system and how to change the direction, if required. The direction of axial slices of the head tend to run inferior to superior, which enables easier comparison with CT head scan slices. Always check the imaging slice direction and anatomical markings are as expected, and according to the local protocol preference. This is especially important when setting up the planes for any joints or extremities (e.g. elbow, hands, or feet). Outstretched hands, for example, are placed in a different anatomical position to the head position, i.e. the body may be 'head-first' but the hand is in a different position when the outstretched limb is above the head. Understand how to enter the patient on the system so that the patient's position has been entered correctly (e.g. prone, supine, head-first, feet- first etc.). This will help to ensure the anatomical markers are correctly displayed on the monitor screen.
Resolution	Defined by the voxel size and a function of FOV and matrix size. Increasing matrix from 128 × 128 to 512 × 512, for example, will offer increased resolution if the FOV is unchanged. However, the SNR will be reduced.
SNR	Affected by FOV, slice thickness, matrix, and NEX/no. of averages. The larger the voxel size, the more signal is available as there are more proton vectors in the sample area. Phase oversampling may provide increased SNR more efficiently than increasing the NEX/no. of averages. Parallel imaging (SENSE/ASSET/ARC/GRAPPA etc.) reduces imaging time but can also reduce SNR. Be aware of any potential reduction in image quality or increase in artefact.

(Continued)

Pulse Sequence Information and Considerations

Consideration	Information/Actions to Consider
Metal Reduction Techniques and Sequences	Use SE or FSE instead of GRE sequences to reduce the signal void from metal in the FOV.
	Increase receiver bandwidth
	Increase spatial resolution
	Do not use interpolation
	Where available, consider using the manufacturer's metal reduction sequences (e.g. MARS, Maverick, OMAR, VAT, SEMAC, etc.).
Radial K-space Filling and Motion Correction Techniques:	Radial k-space filling sequences such as BLADE, Propeller, JET or MultiVane, etc. improve image quality when there is movement in certain directions during the scan.
	Sometimes single shot techniques work well for movement (HASTE/SS-FSE/SSH-TSE/FASE etc.).
Scan Time	For SE, scan time = TR × no. of phase encodings × NEX.
	For FSE, scan time = TR × no. of phase encodings/ETL × NEX.
Reducing SAR	See Table 2.6.

Notes

Notes

5 Preparing for Emergency Situations

Standard Operating Procedures for Dealing with Emergencies

Training to respond to situations requiring urgent attention in MRI requires understanding the consequences of the unique environment. Strong magnetic fields, working within a Faraday cage, and the implications for the MR system if essential requirements such as water or power are not available, make dealing with emergencies in this imaging modality complex.

Having appropriate guidance to follow when something goes wrong may help to ensure that no one is put in a position where they don't know what to do. If the unique operating procedures required to deal with the situation have already been thought through, the resulting processes may enable the best chance of a successful outcome. Guidance, in the form of locally agreed written instructions or SOPs, is recommended and best developed from combined wisdom from those responsible for MR safety. Advice can be sought from the local MR Safety Committee, regulatory bodies, professional bodies and user manuals.

It is also recommended to perform emergency drills/simulations so that everyone is familiar with what to do. This is especially important if the process relates to incidents that are rare events. (See Resources section for more information about SOPs).

Table 5.1 Examples of Scenarios

Emergency or Situation Requiring Urgent Attention	Risks, Response Plan, Location of Guidance
Manual Quench	
Automatic/Spontaneous Quench	
Projectile Incident – large – where someone could be trapped by the object	

(Continued)

Preparing for Emergency Situations

Emergency or Situation Requiring Urgent Attention	Risks, Response Plan, Location of Guidance
Projectile Incident – small – where the object has struck the magnet only or is stuck against the magnet	
Oxygen Monitor Alarming	
Medical Emergency in the Scan Room	
Electrical Power Failure	
Medical Gases Concern (where there is an indication of a problem)	
Fire In or Near the Scan Room	
Violent/Aggressive Patient in the Scan Room or elsewhere in the MR CAA	
Undisclosed Implant/Foreign Body Seen During Scan	
Chemical/QA/QC Phantom Spill	
Flood	

Emergency or Situation Requiring Urgent Attention	Risks, Response Plan, Location of Guidance
Bomb Threat	
Compressor or Chiller Failure	
IT Connectivity Failure	
RF Door Failure	
Air Handling Issue (where a failure of the automatic air extraction system occurs in the scan room or equipment/technical room)	
Telecommunications Failure	
Hydraulic Lift Failure (on mobile scanner)	
Patient Trapped in the Bore (due to faulty table mechanism)	
Patient Stuck at Height on the Table (due to faulty table mechanism)	

Preparing for Emergency Situations

Some General Considerations When Dealing with Emergencies and Urgent Situations in an MRI Department

- What training is provided on how to deal with emergencies?
- Is there a written SOP or guidance document available for each of the potential emergencies listed in Table 5.1, for example?
- How is emergency training for MRI incidents maintained, e.g. are there SOPs on how to perform emergency drills/simulations and if so, how often are drills performed?
- Are MRI safety-trained staff always available to remove someone from the scan room?
- How many staff would likely be required to remove an unconscious patient from the scan room?
- If not using a dockable table, are all emergency MR Conditional trolleys or wheelchairs that are to be used for patient retrieval from the scan room able to support the maximum patient weight limit for the scanner table?
- If the table is dockable, and removed from the scan room with the patient on it, is it safe to defibrillate a patient using electronic defibrillation equipment while the patient is still on the dockable table, i.e. has it been confirmed with the manufacturer that it is safe to do this? If not confirmed by the manufacturer, does this change the management of the situation? What is the local process to be followed?
- At what level of oxygen is the oxygen monitor alarm triggered and what process is followed when it alarms?
- Be aware that an oxygen monitor alarming could also indicate a fault in the alarm system or that a new sensor is required. Is the oxygen monitor regularly serviced? Is the process for investigating what may be the cause for the alarm being set off included in the local guidance?
- Imagine if basic screening fails as well as supervision of the scan room door, and someone brings a large ferrous object, e.g. a wheelchair, into the scan room. If you or someone else becomes trapped by this projectile, how do you call for help? Is there any kind of MRI scan room emergency alert system?
- How do you ensure that any first responders to an emergency in the MRI department will not cause more issues, i.e. if they have not been screened for MRI safety and try to enter the scan room?
- If MRI screening or supervision of who enters the scan room has failed, and someone takes in a ferrous object, how do you prevent this from happening again? Have those tasked with the overall management of staff and patient safety considered implementation of FMDs as a final warning system?
- If the scan room door is open and left unsupervised and someone tries to enter the scan room without being screened, is there any physical barrier across the door frame to act as a final deterrent to entry?
- Are there sufficient and appropriate warning notices and safety interventions in place to alert people of the dangers of entering the scan room unsupervised?
- Consider what issues face a fire team if responding to a fire in or near a superconducting magnet.
- Understand why there is a need to prepare local staff and the fire service on the risks and hazards of dealing with a fire situation in, or near, an MRI scanner.
- How do managers try to ensure that the organisation's fire officer and relevant fire service's fire officer/commander, where appropriate, receive adequate information about the location of any superconducting magnets and the safe processes to follow if responding to a call to the MRI department?

- How can the relevant people learn about the differences between the various types of emergency buttons or switches (quench/magnet rundown, electrical isolation, emergency stop, etc.) that exist in the MRI suite and the consequences of activating such devices?
- Are the medical sockets/outlets, i.e. sockets that provide a backup emergency power supply, easily identified so that critical equipment can always be plugged into the appropriate outlet?
- If there is an electrical power cut, are there MR Conditional torches available or some other way to provide sufficient light to safely evacuate people from the scan room?
- If the scanner has no electrical power, how does this affect the compressor, chiller or the cold head equipment? What are the consequences of no electrical power over a period of time?
- If there is no electrical power to the scan table, how do you remove a non-ambulant patient from the table?
- If there is failure of the compressor or chiller system what are the potential consequences and what should be done?
- If there is damage to the scan room RF door such that it cannot be closed properly, what are the consequences and what should be done?
- Do you know how to quench the magnet, if required, in a situation where there is a risk to life? For example, if someone is pinned to the magnet by a ferrous object.
- Do you know how to contact the scanner manufacturer to alert them to an incident where the magnet needs to be ramped down (i.e. not quenched)? For example, to remove a ferrous object stuck to the magnet where there is no apparent risk to life.

Notes

6 Developing a Protocol for MRI Safety Checks During General Anaesthetic (GA) MRI Sessions

Developing robust protocols and processes may help to prepare a team for the safety interventions required when dealing with anaesthetised, incapacitated and sedated patients. The following suggested system of safety checks is designed to promote a safe working practice.

For those considering introducing anaesthetic sessions, or sedated patient sessions which require anaesthetic support, developing a safety protocol and checklists can help to enable staff to know their role and safety responsibilities during such sessions. Several pauses for checks are required to be performed on any patient's journey from arriving at the MRI department to leaving again. For anaesthetic or incapacitated patients, however, several more checks are required to be introduced. Using a checklist, each stage in the patient's journey into and out of the scan room can be noted to ensure that no checks are missed.

The patient may arrive in the department already anaesthetised, in which case, consent and pre-screening procedures would likely have already been completed and accepted according to local protocol. Alternatively, the patient will arrive at the department to be anaesthetised. Implementing a checklist and creating safety pauses/stops for comprehensive checks of the patient, accompanying staff, carers and all associated equipment, are an important part of this safety initiative. Creating a specific GA MRI safety pathway or workflow is a practical way to ensure that appropriate and sufficient checks are made before the patient or staff enter the scan room. For further guidance on checklists see the Resources section.

Checks performed by MR Authorised person with the lead anaesthetist or anaesthetic team lead before the anaesthetised patient or patient pre-anaesthesia is called to the MRI department. Any initial patient MRI safety are expected to have been have been flagged for investigation at this stage as per local protocol.

- Before the first patient of a GA session is called for, discuss with the GA Team Lead what the patient order and scan order should be, and find out if there are any extra procedures to be performed while any patient on the list is anaesthetised, i.e. any non-MRI investigations such as a lumbar puncture. It may desired that appropriate procedures which are normally performed under GA are to be done while the patient is asleep in the CAA but not in the MR Environment/scan room. Confirm the type of MRI exam to be performed, whether contrast is to be administered and discuss patient positioning requirements and any coil changes.

Knowing the time when breath holds are most crucial for a scan may be useful information for the anaesthetist to ensure adequate breath holds are obtained for those particular scans.

- If the anaesthetist is made aware, for example, that breath holds are required for scanning the abdomen and the patient is having their head scanned too, the anaesthetist may prefer for the abdomen to be scanned first so that the breath holds are performed early.

Check how, or if, MR Conditional transport needs to be sent to the area to collect the patient.

- As per the local policy, check where and how appropriate MR Conditional patient transport is to be used, i.e. if the patient is to be transferred onto MR Conditional transport before arriving at the MRI department from a ward or when they arrive in the MRI department.

Figure 6.1 Some Checks to Consider Before the Patient is Called to the Department.

1st pause and checks performed outside the CAA, typically in either a holding area, waiting area or ward. Performed by appropriate MR Authorised staff before an anaesthetised patient or patient pre-anaesthesia enters the CAA.

1. Patient ID and consent checks performed.
2. Accompanying GA staff ID checks performed.
3. With the GA Team Lead, or as appropriate, confirm the details again of the scan order/exam type to be performed and any extra procedures to be performed when the patient is under GA.
4. Patient MRI safety screening form check performed.
5. As per local process, the patient may require to be changed into MR Safe attire
6. Patient transport check: what the patient arrived on; what they are to be transferred on to; what appropriate MR Conditional or MR Safe patient transport is to be used.
7. If each team member introduces themselves to each other this would ensure that everyone is familiar with each other's role during the session.

2nd pause and checks performed in or out of the CAA as per the department's layout.

MR Authorised person (Supervisor) double-checks that all relevant MRI safety concerns are addressed with the patient/patient's carer/patient's doctor (as appropriate and as per the local SOP) before the patient is anaesthetised. This may involve re-checking/confirming what has been checked at the 1st pause.

3rd pause and checks performed just prior to the patient being taken into the MR Environment/scan room – when the patient is anaesthetised and following pause and checks no.1 and no. 2. More pauses and checks on staff may be required whenever anyone tries to enter the scan room to deal with the patient or to retrieve the patient.

- Once all MRI safety screening checks and any other issues have been adequately addressed, the patient is anaesthetised.
- Patient positioning requirements, any coil changes or plans for giving contrast etc are confirmed again with the anaesthetic team.
- Pre-scan room entry MRI safety checks are then performed by the MR Authorised person (Supervisor) ensuring all MR Unsafe attachments, e.g. ECG sensors, leads, clamps, pumps, pulse oximeters, probes, etc., are either removed or changed to MR Conditional or MR Safe ones.
- Final visual checks are made of the patient's body for any attachments or piercings, and the patient's clothing and hair, as well as any bed sheets or blankets, to ensure no contraindicated items are missed.
- Visual and verbal checks on accompanying GA team members are then performed to check their hair and pockets for any forgotten ferrous items, plus checks to find any other extraneous items they may have about their person such as jewellery, glasses, pens, phones, coins, badges, pagers, etc.
- Final patient transport trolley/gurney checks are made to include visual inspection under sheets, within sheets, on top of trolley, attached to trolley, under trolley.
- Following a checklist on what to check and recording the checks before entering the scan room, may help to avoid missing a contraindicated item. If anyone enters the scan room to deal with the patient (e.g to administer a drug or to retrieve the patient), further pre-entry pauses for checks can be made to mitigate the risk, for example, of someone placing a ferrous item in their pocket by mistake.

Figure 6.2 Some Checks and Pauses to Consider When the Patient Arrives at the MRI Department.

Table 6.1 Further Considerations for MRI GA Sessions – Notes

MR CAA/scan room setup	
Equipment required	
Are there agreed processes to follow during GA or sedated patient sessions?	
What is the process to follow if any stage of the GA safety checks or pauses are breached, i.e. how is a breach of the rules reported and the incident prevented from recurring?	
Communication between the MR and GA team is useful before the list starts, how is this enabled?	
How do the anaesthetic team's MR Authorised personnel maintain such authorisation and how are they signed off as being MRI safety trained?	
What does the GA team's MRI safety training consist of?	
Where are the team's MRI safety training records kept, e.g. local MRI safety training records folder?	
Has an up-to-date MRI staff screening form been completed by the team attending?	
If visiting staff attend to perform procedures on the patient while the patient is under GA, i.e. staff who are not trained in MRI safety, what safety controls are implemented for such staff?	
Consider a coloured lanyard approach so that non-MR staff in the CAA who are MR Authorised wear a lanyard which visually identifies them as safe to enter the scan room (after being previously screened and authorised to enter). This identification process may help to avoid confusion if staff have to enter the scan room in an emergency.	
What is the process for checking if the scan is complete?	
Post procedure considerations	
Consider what processes are to be followed when scanning sedated patients	

Notes

Notes

7 Infection Control Processes

Table 7.1 Infection Prevention and Control Considerations/Notes

Considerations	Information Found at	Notes
Does the MRI screening form or associated information regarding the patient have a question that highlights anything that would result in a change in the normal infection prevention and control measures? How would you, for example, be alerted to the fact that the patient has a communicable disease?		
Is there any alert on the patient's electronic/medical record to indicate infection concerns?		
Process for dealing with a patient that has a communicable disease		
Infection control SOP		
Enhanced cleaning regimes		
General cleaning tasks, checklist, and processes to be followed		
Areas within the MR CAA that may require special care		
Products to be used for scan table and equipment such as coils and padding, as per the manufacturer's recommendations		

(*Continued*)

Infection Control Processes

Considerations	Information Found at	Notes
Authorised/recommended cleaning wipes		
Cleaning solution(s)		
PPE guidance		
Are there MR Safe patient and staff facemasks available, e.g. metal free and of appropriate filtration etc.?		
Gloves (sterile, non-sterile, non-latex, nitrile, etc.)		
Gowns and plastic aprons, shoe covers, etc.		
Process for decontaminating the scan room		
Consider a protocol for scanning any infectious or potentially infectious patients at the end of the list to give appropriate time to clean the area afterwards.		
Process for dealing with contaminated PPE		

Notes

Notes

8 Templates for Recording Protocol Information

Table 8.1 Protocol Table Template

Protocol: **Coil Information:**

Sequence	Orientation	Anatomical Coverage	Slice Thickness	Slice Gap/Space	FOV	Matrix or Other Information	Post Contrast?

Patient Positioning:

Other Comments:

Templates for Recording Protocol Information

Table 8.1a Preparations

Protocol:	
Patient Preparation	**Scan Room Preparation**
Equipment and Supplies	**Contrast Information**
Additional Preparations and Checking Processes, e.g. When is a Radiologist Called to Check the Scans?	**Post-Processing Checking Process and Requirements, e.g. Reformats, MIPs and What Needs to be Sent to PACS, etc.**

Table 8.1 Protocol Table Template

Protocol: **Coil Information:**

Sequence	Orientation	Anatomical Coverage	Slice Thickness	Slice Gap/Space	FOV	Matrix or Other Information	Post Contrast?

Patient Positioning:

Other Comments:

Table 8.1a Preparations

Protocol:	
Patient Preparation	**Scan Room Preparation**
Equipment and Supplies	**Contrast Information**
Additional Preparations and Checking Processes, e.g. When is a Radiologist Called to Check the Scans?	**Post-Processing Checking Process and Requirements, e.g. Reformats, MIPs and What Needs to be Sent to PACS, etc.**

Templates for Recording Protocol Information

Table 8.1 Protocol Table Template

Protocol: Coil Information:

Sequence	Orientation	Anatomical Coverage	Slice Thickness	Slice Gap/Space	FOV	Matrix or Other Information	Post Contrast?

Patient Positioning:

Other Comments:

Templates for Recording Protocol Information

Table 8.1a Preparations

Protocol:	
Patient Preparation	**Scan Room Preparation**
Equipment and Supplies	**Contrast Information**
Additional Preparations and Checking Processes, e.g. When is a Radiologist Called to Check the Scans?	**Post-Processing Checking Process and Requirements, e.g. Reformats, MIPs and What Needs to be Sent to PACS, etc.**

Table 8.2 Emergency Spine Protocol

Protocol: Emergency Spine   Coil Information:

Sequence	Orientation	Anatomical Coverage	Slice Thickness	Slice Gap/Space	FOV	Matrix or Other Information	Post Contrast?

Patient Positioning:

Other Comments:

Templates for Recording Protocol Information

Table 8.2a Emergency Spine Imaging Preparations

Protocol: Emergency Spine	
Patient Preparation	**Scan Room Preparation**
Equipment and Supplies	**Contrast Information**
Additional Preparations and Checking Processes, e.g. When is a Radiologist Called to Check the Scans?	**Post-Processing Checking Process and Requirements, e.g. Reformats, MIPs and What Needs to be Sent to PACS, etc.**

Table 8.3 Neuro/Brain Protocol

Protocol: Head   **Coil Information:**

Sequence	Orientation	Anatomical Coverage	Slice Thickness	Slice Gap/Space	FOV	Matrix or Other Information	Post Contrast?

Patient Positioning:

Other Comments:

Table 8.3a Neuro/Brain Imaging Preparations

Templates for Recording Protocol Information

Protocol: Neuro/Brain	
Patient Preparation	**Scan Room Preparation**
Equipment and Supplies	**Contrast Information**
Additional Preparations and Checking Processes, e.g. When is a Radiologist Called to Check the Scans?	**Post-Processing Checking Process and Requirements, e.g. Reformats, MIPs and What Needs to be Sent to PACS, etc.**

Table 8.4 Musculoskeletal Protocol Table

Protocol: Musculoskeletal   **Coil Information:**

Sequence	Orientation	Anatomical Coverage	Slice Thickness	Slice Gap/Space	FOV	Matrix or Other Information	Post Contrast?

Patient Positioning:

Other Comments:

Templates for Recording Protocol Information

Table 8.4a — Musculoskeletal Imaging Preparations

Protocol: Musculoskeletal	
Patient Preparation	**Scan Room Preparation**
Equipment and Supplies	**Contrast Information**
Additional Preparations and Checking Processes, e.g. When is a Radiologist Called to Check the Scans?	**Post-Processing Checking Process and Requirements, e.g. Reformats, MIPs and What Needs to be Sent to PACS, etc.**

Table 8.5 Angiography Protocol

Protocol: Angiography   **Coil Information:**

Sequence	Orientation	Anatomical Coverage	Slice Thickness	Slice Gap/Space	FOV	Matrix or Other Information	Post Contrast?

Patient Positioning:

Other Comments:

Templates for Recording Protocol Information

Table 8.5a Angiography Imaging Preparations

Protocol: Angiography	
Patient Preparation	**Scan Room Preparation**
Equipment and Supplies	**Contrast Information**
Additional Preparations and Checking Processes, e.g. When is a Radiologist Called to Check the Scans?	**Post-Processing Checking Process and Requirements, e.g. Reformats, MIPs and What Needs to be Sent to PACS, etc.**

Table 8.6 Liver Protocol

Protocol: Liver   **Coil Information:**

Sequence	Orientation	Anatomical Coverage	Slice Thickness	Slice Gap/Space	FOV	Matrix or Other Information	Post Contrast?

Patient Positioning:

Other Comments:

Templates for Recording Protocol Information

| Table 8.6a | Liver Imaging Preparations |

Protocol: Liver	
Patient Preparation	**Scan Room Preparation**
Equipment and Supplies	**Contrast Information**
Additional Preparations and Checking Processes, e.g. When is a Radiologist Called to Check the Scans?	**Post-Processing Checking Process and Requirements, e.g. Reformats, MIPs and What Needs to be Sent to PACS, etc.**

Table 8.7 Small Bowel Imaging/Enterography Protocol

Protocol: Small Bowel/Enterography   **Coil Information:**

Sequence	Orientation	Anatomical Coverage	Slice Thickness	Slice Gap/Space	FOV	Matrix or Other Information	Post Contrast?

Patient Positioning:

Other Comments:

Table 8.7a Small Bowel/Enterography Imaging Preparations

Protocol: Small Bowel/Enterography	
Patient Preparation	**Scan Room Preparation**
Equipment and Supplies	**Contrast Information**
Additional Preparations and Checking Processes, e.g. When is a Radiologist Called to Check the Scans?	**Post-Processing Checking Process and Requirements, e.g. Reformats, MIPs and What Needs to be Sent to PACS, etc.**

Table 8.8 Breast Imaging Protocol

Protocol: Breast Imaging Protocol   Coil Information:

Sequence	Orientation	Anatomical Coverage	Slice Thickness	Slice Gap/Space	FOV	Matrix or Other Information	Post Contrast?

Patient Positioning:

Fat Suppression Method/Spectral Peaks/Curves Information:

Other Comments:

Table 8.8a Breast Imaging Preparations

Protocol: Breast Imaging	
Patient Preparation	**Scan Room Preparation**
Equipment and Supplies	**Contrast Information**
Additional Preparations and Checking Processes, e.g. When is a Radiologist Called to Check the Scans?	**Post-Processing Checking Process and Requirements, e.g. Reformats, MIPs and What Needs to be Sent to PACS, etc.**

Table 8.9 Prostate Imaging Protocol

Protocol: Prostate Imaging **Coil Information:**

Sequence	Orientation	Anatomical Coverage	Slice Thickness	Slice Gap/Space	FOV	Matrix or Other Information	Post Contrast?

Patient Positioning:

Other Comments:

Table 8.9a Prostate Imaging Preparations

Protocol: Prostate	
Patient Preparation	**Scan Room Preparation**
Equipment and Supplies	**Contrast Information**
Additional Preparations and Checking Processes, e.g. When is a Radiologist Called to Check the Scans?	**Post-Processing Checking Process and Requirements, e.g. Reformats, MIPs and What Needs to be Sent to PACS, etc.**

Templates for Recording Protocol Information

Table 8.10 Cardiac Imaging Protocol

Protocol: Cardiac Imaging   Coil Information:

Sequence	Orientation	Anatomical Coverage	Slice Thickness	Slice Gap/Space	FOV	Matrix or Other Information	Post Contrast?

Patient Positioning:

	Short Axis:	Chambers:
	Long Axis:	Chambers:

Other Comments:

Templates for Recording Protocol Information

Table 8.10a Cardiac Imaging Preparations

Protocol: Cardiac Imaging	
Patient Preparation	**Scan Room Preparation**
Equipment and Supplies	**Contrast Information**
Additional Preparations and Checking Processes, e.g. When is a Radiologist Called to Check the Scans?	**Post-Processing Checking Process and Requirements, e.g. Reformats, MIPs and What Needs to be Sent to PACS, etc.**

Table 8.11 Whole Body Imaging Protocol

Protocol: Whole Body Imaging **Coil Information:**

Sequence	Orientation	Anatomical Coverage	Slice Thickness	Slice Gap/Space	FOV	Matrix or Other Information	Post Contrast?

Patient Positioning:

Other Comments:

Templates for Recording Protocol Information

Table 8.11a Whole Body Imaging Preparations

Protocol: Whole Body	
Patient Preparation	**Scan Room Preparation**
Equipment and Supplies	**Contrast Information**
Additional Preparations and Checking Processes, e.g. When is a Radiologist Called to Check the Scans?	**Post-Processing Checking Process and Requirements, e.g. Reformats, MIPs and What Needs to be Sent to PACS, etc.**

Table 8.12 Paediatric Imaging Protocol

Protocol: Paediatric Imaging　　　　Coil Information:

Sequence	Orientation	Anatomical Coverage	Slice Thickness	Slice Gap/Space	FOV	Matrix or Other Information	Post Contrast?

Patient Positioning:

Other Comments:

Table 8.12a Paediatric Imaging Preparations

Protocol: Paediatric	
Patient Preparation	**Scan Room Preparation**
Equipment and Supplies	**Contrast Information**
Additional Preparations and Checking Processes, e.g. When is a Radiologist Called to Check the Scans?	**Post-Processing Checking Process and Requirements, e.g. Reformats, MIPs and What Needs to be Sent to PACS, etc.**

Templates for Recording Protocol Information

Table 8.12 Paediatric Imaging Protocol

Protocol: Paediatric Imaging — **Coil Information:**

Sequence	Orientation	Anatomical Coverage	Slice Thickness	Slice Gap/ Space	FOV	Matrix or Other Information	Post Contrast?

Patient Positioning:

Other Comments:

Templates for Recording Protocol Information

Table 8.12a Paediatric Imaging Preparations

Protocol: Paediatric	
Patient Preparation	**Scan Room Preparation**
Equipment and Supplies	**Contrast Information**
Additional Preparations and Checking Processes, e.g. When is a Radiologist Called to Check the Scans?	**Post-Processing Checking Process and Requirements, e.g. Reformats, MIPs and What Needs to be Sent to PACS, etc.**

Table 8.12 Paediatric Imaging Protocol

Protocol: Paediatric Imaging   Coil Information:

Sequence	Orientation	Anatomical Coverage	Slice Thickness	Slice Gap/Space	FOV	Matrix or Other Information	Post Contrast?

Patient Positioning:

Other Comments:

Table 8.12a Paediatric Imaging Preparations

Protocol: Paediatric	
Patient Preparation	**Scan Room Preparation**
Equipment and Supplies	**Contrast Information**
Additional Preparations and Checking Processes, e.g. When is a Radiologist Called to Check the Scans?	**Post-Processing Checking Process and Requirements, e.g. Reformats, MIPs and What Needs to be Sent to PACS, etc.**

Templates for Recording Protocol Information

Table 8.12 Paediatric Imaging Protocol

Protocol: Paediatric Imaging   Coil Information:

Sequence	Orientation	Anatomical Coverage	Slice Thickness	Slice Gap/Space	FOV	Matrix or Other Information	Post Contrast?

Patient Positioning:

Other Comments:

Table 8.12a Paediatric Imaging Preparations

Protocol: Paediatric	
Patient Preparation	**Scan Room Preparation**
Equipment and Supplies	**Contrast Information**
Additional Preparations and Checking Processes, e.g. When is a Radiologist Called to Check the Scans?	**Post-Processing Checking Process and Requirements, e.g. Reformats, MIPs and What Needs to be Sent to PACS, etc.**

Table 8.13 Active Research Projects Protocols

Protocol: Active Research Projects **Coil Information:**

Sequence	Orientation	Anatomical Coverage	Slice Thickness	Slice Gap/Space	FOV	Matrix or Other Information	Post Contrast?

Patient Positioning:

Other Comments:

Templates for Recording Protocol Information

Table 8.13a Active Research Projects Preparations

Protocol: Active Research Projects	
Patient Preparation	**Scan Room Preparation**
Equipment and Supplies	**Contrast Information**
Additional Preparations and Checking Processes, e.g. When is a Radiologist Called to Check the Scans?	**Post-Processing Checking Process and Requirements, e.g. Reformats, MIPs and What Needs to be Sent to PACS, etc.**

Table 8.14 Escalation Process If Pathology Seen

Escalation Process if Pathology Seen (Who to contact and how)	Policy for Escalation Process if Out of Normal Working Hours

Notes

9 Contrast Considerations

Follow local policy on how to deal with an adverse contrast/drug reaction and an extravasation event.

Table 9.1 Adverse Contrast/Drug Reaction Considerations

Considerations	Dealing with an Adult Drug Reaction	Dealing with a Paediatric Drug Reaction	How to Deal with an Extravasation
Immediate action plan			
How to ensure the patient is in a safe area for treatment			
Emergency Response Team contact information and what should be stated when calling			
How to ensure emergency responders (if not screened for MRI safety) do not enter the scan room			
Location of appropriate crash/emergency trolley and any other emergency equipment such as anaphylaxis kit, oxygen cylinder, suction, defibrillator, etc.			
How and when training is provided for dealing with such situations, as per the local SOP			
Documentation required post event: where and how to report the adverse event. Is it reported to local/national reporting systems, as well as to the manufacturer? Is there any additional process to follow to check on the patient's condition after they have left the department?			

Table 9.2 eGFR and Creatinine Notes

eGFR and Creatinine Notes	
When is an eGFR performed and on what types of patients?	
Where do you find instructions on how to use the Point-of-Care Device for Measuring Creatinine (as per local process)?	
Where to locate the Point-of-Care Device	
According to the local policy, what eGFR value is required to inject gadolinium based contrast?	
Where to record the findings	
What is the process if the eGFR does not reach the criteria required?	

Table 9.3 Contrast Injection Considerations for Patients with Additional Needs

Considerations for Those with Additional Needs Who Require Contrast	
Location of local process to follow and what documentation is to be recorded	
What processes are in place?	
What trained staff can be called upon to assist? Are there any specialist nurses who are trained in dealing with patients with heightened anxieties, phobias or learning difficulties and is there a play therapist available to help to relax a child for their injection?	
What environmental changes can help?	
What equipment/distractions can help?	
What training is provided?	

Table 9.4 Other Processes to Consider	
Other Processes to Consider	
What if the patient refuses contrast or other drug, e.g. Buscopan?	
Location of local process to follow and what documentation is to be recorded	
Action plan, i.e. alternative	
What trained staff can be called for advice/to assist?	
Remember to amend any annotation on the images/RIS/PACS system if the expected contrast administration does not take place	
What is the process to follow if venous access is difficult?	
Location of local process to follow and what documentation is to be recorded	
Is there a phlebotomist or clinician available who can try to inject, as per the local procedures?	
What is the process to follow if the patient is pregnant or lactating?	
Location of local process to follow and what documentation is to be recorded	

Please follow guidelines from the manufacturer and your local processes for administration of any contrast or other drugs as per your organisation's policies.

Table 9.5 Template of Contrast or Other Drug Administration Notes

Name of contrast agent or other drug:	
Method of delivery (pump/hand injection/oral/nasogastric/intracavity):	
Method/formula for calculating the dose/amount to be administered:	Indication and usage:
Saline flush volume (if relevant):	Checks and vigilance to be undertaken before pumping contrast:
Contrast or drug manufacturer's contact and website details:	
Injection or delivery flow rate:	Contraindication and precautions:
Pump injection details:	Post-contrast checks to be made on the patient and how long they are required to remain in the department:
Post-scan check of requirement to recharge injector pump batteries:	
Notes:	

Contrast Considerations

Table 9.5 Template of Contrast or Other Drug Administration Notes

Name of contrast agent or other drug:	
Method of delivery (pump/hand injection/oral/nasogastric/intracavity):	
Method/formula for calculating the dose/amount to be administered:	Indication and usage:
Saline flush volume (if relevant):	Checks and vigilance to be considered before pumping contrast:
Contrast or drug manufacturer's contact and website details:	
Injection or delivery flow rate:	Contraindication and precautions:
Pump injection details:	Post-contrast checks to be made on the patient (as per local policy e.g. how long the patient remains in the department and what checks are performed):
Post-scan check of requirement to recharge injector pump batteries:	
Notes:	

Contrast Considerations

Table 9.5 Template of Contrast or Other Drug Administration Notes

Name of contrast agent or other drug:	
Method of delivery (pump/hand injection/oral/nasogastric/intracavity):	
Method/formula for calculating the dose/amount to be administered:	Indication and usage:
Saline flush volume (if relevant):	Checks and vigilance to be undertaken before pumping contrast:
Contrast or drug manufacturer's contact and website details:	
Injection or delivery flow rate:	Contraindication and precautions:
Pump injection details:	Post-contrast checks to be made on the patient and how long they are required to remain in the department:
Post-scan check of requirement to recharge injector pump batteries:	
Notes:	

Table 9.5 Template of Contrast or Other Drug Administration Notes

Name of contrast agent or other drug:	
Method of delivery (pump/hand injection/oral/nasogastric/intracavity):	
Method/formula for calculating the dose/amount to be administered:	Indication and usage:
Saline flush volume (if relevant):	Checks and vigilance to be undertaken before pumping contrast:
Contrast or drug manufacturer's contact and website details:	
Injection or delivery flow rate:	Contraindication and precautions:
Pump injection details:	Post-contrast checks to be made on the patient and how long they are required to remain in the department:
Post-scan check of requirement to recharge injector pump batteries:	
Notes:	

Table 9.5 Template of Contrast or Other Drug Administration Notes

Name of contrast agent or other drug:	
Method of delivery (pump/hand injection/oral/nasogastric/intracavity):	
Method/formula for calculating the dose/amount to be administered:	Indication and usage:
Saline flush volume (if relevant):	Checks and vigilance to be undertaken before pumping contrast:
Contrast or drug manufacturer's contact and website details:	
Injection or delivery flow rate:	Contraindication and precautions:
Pump injection details:	Post-contrast checks to be made on the patient and how long they are required to remain in the department:
Post-scan check of requirement to recharge injector pump batteries:	
Notes:	

Table 9.5 Template of Contrast or Other Drug Administration Notes

Name of contrast agent or other drug:	
Method of delivery (pump/hand injection/oral/nasogastric/intracavity):	
Method/formula for calculating the dose/amount to be administered:	Indication and usage:
Saline flush volume (if relevant):	Checks and vigilance to be undertaken before pumping contrast:
Contrast or drug manufacturer's contact and website details:	
Injection or delivery flow rate:	Contraindication and precautions:
Pump injection details:	Post-contrast checks to be made on the patient and how long they are required to remain in the department:
Post-scan check of requirement to recharge injector pump batteries:	
Notes:	

Notes

10 Image Artefact Considerations

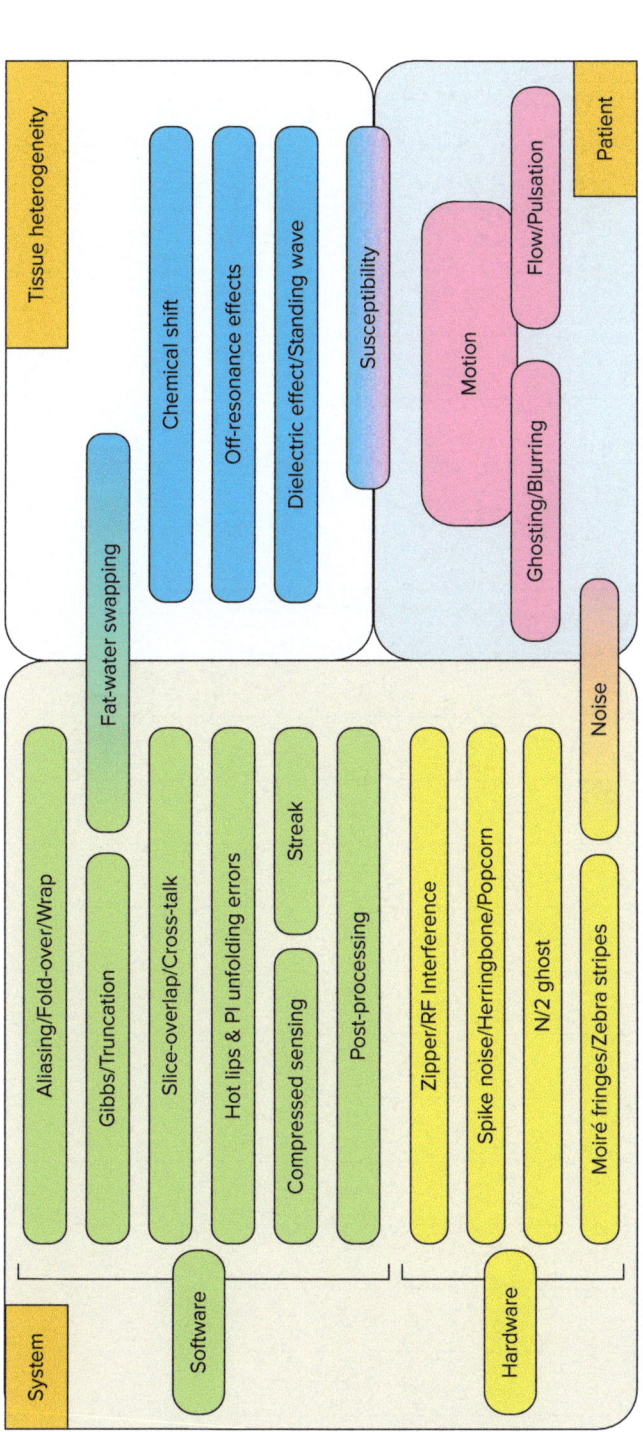

Figure 10.1 Depiction of Typical MRI Image Artefacts.

PI = parallel imaging, *RF* = radiofrequency

Noda, C., Ambale-Venkatesh, B., Wagner, J. D., Kato, Y., Ortman, J., & Lima, J. A. (2022). Primer on commonly occurring MRI artifacts and how to overcome them. *Radiographics*, 42(3), E102–E103. https://doi.org/10.1148/rg.210021

For some suggested reading about artefacts, see Resources section.

Notes

11 Miscellaneous Topics and Concerns

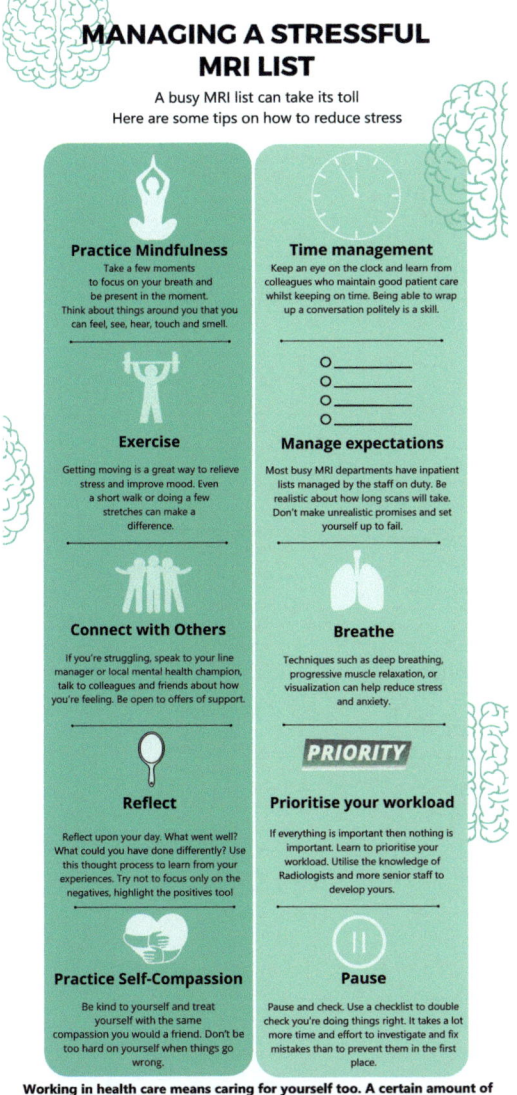

Figure 11.1 Managing a Stressful List, template design. ©colllabsupply via Canva.com

See Resources Section for organisations to contact for support.

Table 11.1 Additional Topics to Consider

Additional Topics to Consider	Location of Guidance / Notes
Breast implants	
Dermal piercings	
'Electromagnetic Hypersensitivity' belief – where patient may be wearing what's sold as 'EMF-Shielded' clothing and this contains metal (hats, underwear etc.).	
External fixation systems	
Eyelid weights	
GISP	
Incident reporting: how, what and why to report safety incidents and the importance of reporting 'near-miss' events (where no one was hurt or equipment damaged but it might happen again).	
IOFB	
Lactating patients and contrast considerations	
Lactating and/or menstruating patients if underwear is to be removed (provisions for patient comfort, hygiene and dignity)	

Miscellaneous Topics and Concerns

Additional Topics to Consider	Location of Guidance / Notes
Use of Melatonin to induce sleep in very young children, to enable them to be scanned without GA. (Note that the appropriate medical/anaesthetic team would be involved.)	
'Feed and wrap' methods to scan babies in natural sleep	
Cosmetic procedures and enhancements that may involve (semi-)permanent ink containing metal particles, e.g. micro-bladed eyebrows, eyeliner, lip liner. Also be aware of the use of magnetic eyelashes.	
Patient information: consider including links to suitable videos showing what to expect when attending for a scan. Can anxious and young patients be given an opportunity to book a pre-visit to encourage compliance?	
Pregnant patients	
Tattoos and other types of body art	
Patients with reduced thermoregulatory capacity	
Breast tissue expanders	
Gastric pacemaker	

(Continued)

Miscellaneous Topics and Concerns

Additional Topics to Consider	Location of Guidance / Notes
Stimulators	
Implantable infusion pump	
Aneurysm clip	
Fitness trackers, including smart rings	
Hair extensions	
Precautions required when using laser lights	
Latex allergy – does the patient call-button (or bulb or buzzer) contain latex? (If so, could, for example, a non-latex glove be used to cover it?)	
Penile implants	
The administration of an injectable medicine supplied under a Patient Group Direction (PGD). See NICE guidelines https://www.nice.org.uk/guidance/mpg2 and SoR guidance:https://www.sor.org/news/ezine/new-guide-on-safe-use-of-pgds-in-contrast-media-(1	
Process to deal with a patient burn	

Notes

Notes

12 Recording Continuing Professional Development (CPD)

The Health and Care Professions Council set out the standards of CPD they expect of registrants (https://www.hcpc-uk.org/standards/standards-of-continuing-professional-development/). **The Society of Radiographers' definition of CPD is:** *"An ongoing professional activity in which the practitioner identifies, undertakes and evaluates learning appropriate to the maintenance and development of the highest standards of practice within an evolving scope of practice"* (https://www.sor.org/learning-advice/learning/cpd/cpd-policy-and-guidance).

Have a structured way to evidence a representative sample of your learning activities to demonstrate compliance with your profession's definition of CPD. By describing and undertaking appropriate learning activities and the subsequent learning achieved, your CPD portfolio should demonstrate the actual or intended impact on clinical practice.

Recording Continuing Professional Development (CPD)

Table 12.1 A Template to Note CPD Activities

Types of Activities that may Count as CPD	Examples	CPD Activity	Date	How it Shows Maintenance of Appropriate Standards of Practice
Work based	In-service training; supervising; role extension; applications training; learning a new protocol/procedure; completing self-assessment questionnaires; being on a committee.			
Professional activity	Teaching, mentoring; being involved in a professional body; presenting at a conference; maintaining or developing specialist skills.			
Formal education	Attending conferences; seminars			
	Conducting research; writing articles/papers; presenting your work.			
Self-directed learning	Reading relevant journals, articles, books; keeping a file of your progress; updating your knowledge through the internet or asking experts for advice.			
Reflective practice	Reflecting on experiences at work, considering feedback from patients and colleagues, discussing relevant techniques or processes.			
Other	Relevant public service or voluntary work.			

Notes

Notes

13 Resources

Administration of Contrast Guidance

Bayer https://radiology.bayer.co.uk/

Bracco https://www.bracco.com/en-gb/mri and https://www.bracco.com/en-gb/e-learning

GE Healthcare https://www.gehealthcare.co.uk/products/contrast-media

Guerbet https://www.guerbet.com/en-gb/healthcare-professionals/about-us/guerbet-uk

Royal College of Radiologists Guidance on gadolinium-based contrast agent administration to adult patients | https://www.rcr.ac.uk/our-services/all-our-publications/clinical-radiology-publications/guidance-on-gadolinium-based-contrast-agent-administration-to-adult-patients/

Society of Radiographers Update for radiographers administering contrast agents using a patient group direction | https://www.sor.org/news/contrast-media-and-drugs/update-for-radiographers-administering-contrast-ag

Anaesthesia MRI Checklists and Guidance

World Health Organisation Surgical Safety Checklist Implementation https://www.who.int/teams/integrated-health-services/patient-safety/research/safe-surgery/tool-and-resources.

The British Institute of Radiology MR Safety Advice 2023 mr_advice_sheet_2_safety_steps_in_an_anaesthesia_service_in_the_mri_suite_v2.pdf (bir.org.uk)

Association of Anaesthetists Guidelines – Safe provision of anaesthesia in magnetic resonance units 2019 | https://anaesthetists.org/Home/Resources-publications/Guidelines/Safe-provision-of-anaesthesia-in-magnetic-resonance-units https://anaesthetists.org/

Medicines & Healthcare products Regulatory Agency 4.14 Anaesthesia https://www.gov.uk/government/publications/safety-guidelines-for-magnetic-resonance-imaging-equipment-in-clinical-use

Antenatal and Fetal MRI

American Journal of Roentgenology Malamateniou C, et al. (2013) Motion-compensation techniques in neonatal and fetal MR imaging. AJNR Am J Neuroradiol. 2013 Jun-Jul;34(6):1124-36. doi: 10.3174/ajnr.A3128. Epub 2012 May 10. PMID: 22576885

Handbook Clinical Neurology. Fetal and neonatal neuroimaging.Counsell SJ, et al. 2019;162:67-103. doi: 10.1016/B978-0-444-64029-1.00004-7.PMID: 31324329

Magnetic Resonance Imaging Clinics of North America (2021) Stout JN et al. Fetal Neuroimaging Updates. Nov;29(4):557-581. doi: 10.1016/j.mric.2021.06.007.PMID: 34717845

RAD Magazine Fetal MRI: a practical guide Barbara Nugent, Dr Christina Malamateniou | https://www.radmagazine.com/scientific-article/fetal-mri-a-practical-guide/

Artefacts

American Journal of Roentgenology Hakky M, et al. (2013). Application of basic physics principles to clinical neuroradiology: differentiating artifacts from true pathology on MRI. Am J Roentgenol, 201(2):369–377.

Polish Journal of Radiology Krupa K, Bekiesińska-Figatowska M (2015). Artifacts in magnetic resonance imaging. Pol J Radiol, Feb 23;80:93–106. doi: 10.12659/PJR.892628. PMID: 25745524; PMCID: PMC4340093.

RadioGraphics Primer on Commonly Occurring MRI Artifacts and How to Overcome Them Noda C, et al. RadioGraphics 2022;42(3):E102–E103.

Autism/Neurodiversity Information

Autism Stogiannos et al. (2022). A systematic review of person-centred adjustments to facilitate magnetic resonance imaging for autistic patients without the use of sedation or anaesthesia. Autism, 26(4):782–797. https://doi.org/10.1177/13623613211065542.

Autism in Adulthood Stogiannos N, et al. (2023) Toward autism-friendly magnetic resonance imaging: exploring autistic individuals' experiences of magnetic resonance imaging scans in the United Kingdom, a cross-sectional survey. Autism in Adulthood, 5(3):248–262.

Development Cognitive Neuroscience Pua et al. (2020). Individualised MRI training for paediatric neuroimaging: a child-focused approach. Dev Cogn Neurosci, 41:100750.

Cauda Equina Syndrome Information

RAD Magazine Guidance on MRI provision for cauda equina syndrome. Rachel Watt. | https://www.radmagazine.com/scientific-article/guidance-on-mri-provision-for-cauda-equina-syndrome/

Royal College of Radiologists MRI Provision for Cauda Equina Syndrome | https://www.rcr.ac.uk/our-services/all-our-publications/clinical-radiology-publications/mri-provision-for-cauda-equina-syndrome/ and (IPEM/ SoR/CoR/) | https: /www.ipem.ac.uk/media/dhtmspu3/cib-mri-cauda-equina-syndrome-feb-2023.pdf

Generic Implant Safety Procedures

The British Institute of Radiology, MR Safety Advice 2023, Generic Implant Safety Procedures in MRI: Should we always identify make/model before scanning? https://www.bir.org.uk/media/525500/mr_advice_sheet_3_generic_implant_safety_procedures_in_mri._final.pdf

Manufacturers' Websites

Canon Medical Systems https://uk.medical.canon/products/magnetic-resonance/

Esaote https://www2.esaote.com/magnetic-resonance/education/ and https://www2.esaote.com/magnetic-resonance/technologies/

Fujifilm https://www.fujifilm.com/uk/en/healthcare (or UK),
https://www.fujifilm.com/de/en/healthcare (for Europe)

GE Healthcare weconnect.gehealthcare.com

Philips Healthcare https://www.philips.co.uk/healthcare and https://www.mriclinicalcasemap.

Siemens magnetomworld.siemens-healthineers.com and https://www.magnetomworld.siemens-healthineers.com/publications/mr-basics

MRI Safety, MRI Scanning and MRI Physics Resources

American College of Radiology https://www.acr.org/Clinical-Resources/Radiology-Safety/MR-Safety

American College of Radiology, Committee on MR Safety:; Greenberg TD, et al ACR guidance document on MR safe practices: Updates and critical information 2019. J Magn Reson Imaging. 2020 Feb;51(2):331-338. doi: 10.1002/jmri.26880. Epub 2019 Jul 29. PMID: 31355502.

British Association of Magnetic Resonance Radiographers https://www.BAMRR.org

British Institute of Radiology https://www.bir.org.uk

elfh elearning for healthcare NHS England https://www.e-lfh.org.uk/programmes/all-our-health/ | UK online MRI Safety Training Programme available for free for NHS staff and appropriate institutions in the UK at: https://www.e-lfh.org.uk/programmes/mri-safety/ – or can be purchased at: https://www.eintegrity.org/healthcare-course/mri-safety/

Institute of Physics and Engineering in Medicine (IPEM) https://www.ipem.ac.uk

International Society for MR Radiographers & Technologists https://www.ismrm.org/smrt/

Kanal, E. (2020). Standardized Approaches to MR Safety Assessment of Patients with Implanted Devices. *Magnetic Resonance Imaging Clinics of North America*, 28(4), 537–548. doi: 10.1016/j.mric.2020.07.003

Lipton M Lectures by Dr Michael Lipton, Einstein College of Medicine.

McRobbie DW Essentials of MRI Safety. John Wiley & Sons, 2020.

McRobbie DW, Moore EA, Graves MJ, Prince MR MRI from Picture to Proton, third edition. Cambridge University Press; 2017: iii–iii.

Medicines & Healthcare products Regulatory Agency https://www.gov.uk/government/publications/safety-guidelines-for-magnetic-resonance-imaging-equipment-in-clinical-use

MRI Master.com https://mrimaster.com/

MRI Questions.com https://www.mriquestions.com/index.html

Radiology Assistant https://radiologyassistant.nl/

Radiopaedia https://radiopaedia.org/

Royal College of Radiologists https://www.rcr.ac.uk/

Shellock FG, Crues JV, Karacozoff AM MRI Bioeffects, Safety, and Patient Management 2nd Edition | www.MRIsafetybook.com

Shellock FG http://mrisafety.com/

Society of Radiographers https://www.sor.org

Westbrook C, Talbot J MRI in Practice Course and The Handbook of MRI Technique http://www.mrieducation.com/

Person-Centred Care

British Medical Journal Staniszewska et al. (2017). GRIPP2 reporting checklists: tools to improve reporting of patient and public involvement in research. BMJ, 358 doi: https://doi.org/10.1136/bmj.j3453 (Published 02 August 2017). https://www.bmj.com/content/bmj/358/bmj.j3453.full.pdf

Care Quality Commission Deprivation of Liberty Safeguards (DoLS) https://www.cqc.org.uk/publications/major-report/state-care/2022-2023/dols

Journal of Radiology Nursing Hudson DM, Evans R (2023). A service evaluation of what satisfies our patients in magnetic resonance imaging. J Radiol Nurs, https://doi.org/10.1016/j.jradnu.2023.07.007.

Medical Imaging in Practice Hewis J, Strachan K (2024). Person-centered care in magnetic resonance imaging. In Chau et al. (eds.), Person-Centered Care in Radiology: International Perspectives on High-Quality Care (1st ed.). CRC Press.

National Institute for Health and Care Research PPI (Patient and Public Involvement) resources for applicants to NIHR research programmes | https://www.nihr.ac.uk/documents/ppi-patient-and-public-involvement-resources-for-applicants-to-nihr-research-programmes/23437

Shorrock S Blog: Humanistic Systems | https://humanisticsystems.com/

Strudwick et al. Person-centred Care in Radiography: Skills for Providing Effective Patient Care. Wiley.

Quality Standards

National Occupational Standard HCS MR1. Skills for Health Roles Directory https://tools.skillsforhealth.org.uk/roles-directory/

The College of Radiographers and the Royal College of Radiologists Joint Quality Standards for Imaging https://www.rcr.ac.uk/our-services/management-service-delivery/quality-standard-for-imaging-qsi/

Society and College of Radiographers Code of Professional Conduct: https://www.sor.org/learning-advice/professional-body-guidance-and-publications/documents-and-publications/policy-guidance-document-library/code-of-professional-conduct

UKAS Imaging Services Accreditation https://www.ukas.com/accreditation/standards/quality-standard-imaging/

Health & Care Professions Council (HPCP) https://www.hcpc-uk.org/registration/

HCPC Standards of Conduct, Performance and Ethics https://www.hcpc-uk.org/standards/standards-of-conduct-performance-and-ethics/

Reporting Incidents

MHRA Yellow Card Scheme https://yellowcard.mhra.gov.uk/

SAR Information

International Society for Magnetic Resonance in Medicine Faulkner W (2016). New MRI safety labels and devices. Signals, 5(1) Retrieved from February 2016 issue of "Signals", produced by the International Society for Magnetic Resonance in Medicine (ISMRM) | https://www.ismrm.org/smrt/E-Signals/2016FEBRUARY/eSig_5_1_hot_2.htm

MRI Questions.Com What is B1+rms? Is it a better metric for energy deposition than SAR? | https://mriquestions.com/b1rms-vs-sar.html

Public Health England: https://www.gov.uk/government/publications/magnetic-resonance-imaging-mri-protecting-patients

Additional Information Related to Content

Society of Radiographers 'Have you paused and checked' poster available to download alongside a prompt card | https://www.sor.org/learning-advice/professional-body-guidance-and-publications/documents-and-publications/posters/have-you-paused-and-checked-ir(me)r-posters

College of Radiographers' (CoR) Education and Career Framework (provides guidance for the education and career development of the radiography profession)

https://www.sor.org/learning-advice/professional-body-guidance-and-publications/documents-and-publications/policy-guidance-document-library/education-and-career-framework-fourth

SOP information from NHS Education for Scotland, Human Factors Hub: https://learn.nes.nhs.scot/30397

General points to consider over accountability in the UK from the Society of Radiographers

Employers'/Organisations' Responsibilities

Employers have a responsibility to ensure that a safe service is in place for patients and staff and should have specific frameworks to ensure appropriate training, education, competencies and skill mix are developed. The framework should set out clearly the roles and responsibilities of employees.

The College of Radiographers and the Royal College of Radiologists have published the Quality Standard for Imaging (see link in Quality Standards section above) which sets out the expectations for delivery of a quality service and includes governance and leadership standards.

Individual Practitioner's Responsibilities

If the scan operator is an HCPC registered practitioner, they are accountable for their actions and are considered responsible for the episode of patient care. Responsibilities and expectations are set out in the HCPC Standards of Conduct, Performance and Ethics (see link in Quality Standards section above).

The Society of Radiographers is the professional body for the radiographic workforce in the UK. Its Code of Professional Conduct sets out expectations for an individual's conduct in practice (see link in Quality Standards section above).

Assistant Practitioner Responsibilities

If the scan operator is an assistant practitioner and so not registered with the HCPC, they should be working under a clearly defined scope of practice within a supervision framework.

Further details on governance arrangements, supervision and delegation can be found at: https://www.sor.org/learning-advice/professional-body-guidance-and-publications/documents-and-publications/policy-guidance-document-library/the-radiography-support-and-assistant-workforce-re

If an incident occurs

This should be reported immediately following both the local policy and required regulatory reporting mechanisms.

MRI Contrast Agent Manufacturers' Websites/Educational Resources

1. Bayer: https://radiology.bayer.co.uk/

2. Bracco: https://www.bracco.com/en-gb/e-learning

3. GE Healthcare: https://www.gehealthcare.co.uk/products/contrast-media

4. Guerbet: https://www.guerbet.com/en-gb/healthcare-professionals/about-us/guerbet-uk

MRI Scanner Manufacturers' Websites/Educational Resources

1. Canon Medical Systems: https://uk.medical.canon/products/magnetic-resonance/

2. Esaote: https://www2.esaote.com/magnetic-resonance/education/

3. Fujifilm: https://www.fujifilm.com/uk/en/healthcare

4. GE Healthcare: https://weconnect.gehealthcare.com/

5. Philips Healthcare: https://www.philips.co.uk/healthcare

6. Siemens Healthineers: https://www.magnetomworld.siemens-healthineers.com/

Siemens Healthineers:https://www.magnetomworld.siemens-healthineers.com/publications/mr-basics